Hot Women, Cool Solutions™

Control your menopause symptoms using mind/body techniques'

Pat Duckworth

Published by

HWCS Publications

White House, Meeting Lane

Litlington

Royston, Cambs

England SG8 0QF

The author has done her best to present accurate and up-to-date information in this book, but she cannot guarantee that the information is correct or will suit your particular situation.

Limit of Liability and Disclaimer of Warranty: The publisher has used best efforts in preparing this book, and the information provided herein is provided "as is".

Medical Liability Disclaimer: This book is sold with the understanding that the publisher and the author are not engaged in rendering any legal, medical or any other professional services. If expert assistance is required, the services of a competent professional should be sought.

Cover Design: Max Caddick

For inquiries about volume orders, contact the publisher.

Email pat@patduckworth.com

ISBN: 978-0-9926620-4-2

DEDICATION

To the two Alex Duckworths in my life – my husband
and my son.

FOREWORD

As a coach I am committed to helping people to achieve their goals not only in their work life but also in their personal life. So now, I'd ask you, dear reader, how do you want the rest of your life to be? If you are a woman entering your 40's or 50's you potentially have 40 or more years ahead of you and they can be the best years of your life. To do this you need to start by being well-informed and then take action.

For women approaching menopause there seems to be a stark choice between taking hormone replacement therapy (HRT) or suffering in silence. In American a large proportion of women opt for taking HRT although in the UK the percentage is less but still significant. Since HRT first became available in the late 1940s it has been viewed variously as anything from the magic answer to ageing to a high risk drug treatment.

The decision whether to take HRT is not clear cut and there are other effective options to dealing with menopause symptoms. In this book, Pat Duckworth gives women the information they need to take control of their health and their life and make informed decisions about their own treatment.

The human mind is a powerful tool that can bring about real chemical and physical changes in the brain and the body. There are many neuro-linguistic programming books but Hot Women, Cool Solutions ™ is written by a woman for women. Pat draws from her personal experiences and from her work as a cognitive hypnotherapist working with many women clients. She explains how to use NLP tools in a way that is a pleasure to read and easy to practice.

Whether you are a woman approaching menopause or going through it, this book will inspire you to take a positive approach to this natural stage in your life.

Raymond Aaron

NY Times Bestselling Author

www.UltimateAuthorBootcamp.com

ACKNOWLEDGEMENTS

I was inspired to write this book during my cognitive hypnotherapy graduation weekend at the Quest Institute. Many thanks to Trevor Silvester for that inspiration.

Thanks to my more experienced colleague and friend Patricia McBride for all of her excellent ideas.

Special thanks to all of the women who shared their experiences with me. I have changed their names to protect the innocent but ladies – you know who you are!

CONTENTS

INTRODUCTION

At the time of writing this second edition of 'Hot Women, Cool Solutions', I am pleased to say that the issue of menopause is being more freely and openly discussed than it was in 2012 when the first edition was published. Many celebrity women have stepped forward to share their experiences and workplace menopause is being taken more seriously by employers.

That doesn't mean that everything in the garden is rosy. Most of the language around menopause is still very negative and there is a lingering taboo around talking about it. Many women seem to be reluctant to become informed on the subject until they start experiencing symptoms and wonder what on earth is happening to them.

Let's face it, if you're a woman you know you have to go through the menopause sooner or later. How good would it be if you could use your mind to control your symptoms? Well you can and I'm going to share with you how.

As a cognitive hypnotherapist I have worked with many women clients on a range of issues including poor sleep, weight loss, low mood, lack of confidence, and hot flashes. These can all be indicators of the menopause but few clients have specifically come to me mentioning the 'M' word. Is that because talking about menopause or seeking help with it is still a bit of a taboo? Is it because it's a 'woman's problem' or is it seen negatively as a sign of ageing?

Whatever the reason, I want to start talking about it and helping other women to share their experiences in a positive way. This is just another phase in our lives and it can be the best phase. Given that we are all living longer you may have over forty years of post-menopausal life to enjoy so let's get on with it.

I also want to share some highly effective practical mind/body techniques to control menopausal symptoms. In recent years there has been lots more research published into the powerful effect the mind can have in healing the body (Hamilton 2008). Visualisation has been used in a variety of circumstances not only to improve sports performance but also to help people with a range of medical conditions including arthritis, stroke and spinal injuries. It is amazing how just by visualising a part of your body working well, you can start to re-programme your brain to help it happen.

My aim in writing this book is to help women to approach this period of change in their life positively. If you survived the hormonal turmoil of puberty and the many changes to your body and emotions during that stage of your life, you can definitely be in control during your menopause.

Menopause is not an illness. It is a natural phase of a woman's life and there are lots of actions that you can take to ensure that you stay healthy and fit. The clients I work with learn more about how their mind can affect their body and learn techniques to enable their mind to change and control physical symptoms.

This book is primarily for women in the perimenopause stage of life but if you are younger and you want to stay healthy into your later life read on! The healthier you are going into the menopause, the fitter you will be coming out of the other side. Who doesn't want to be physically and mentally healthy during their retirement and later life?

In this book you will learn more about the symptoms associated with the menopause. I will provide some basic information on good nutrition and exercise and practical tips on lifestyle. I'll also be exploring mind/body techniques that are easy to learn and effective in reducing symptoms and enhancing your mood.

Although I have written this book from a woman's perspective, the lifestyle and diet advice and the techniques are equally applicable to men.

I have added a bonus chapter in this edition, 'Why Menopause is a Workplace Issue' which is taken from my most recent book, 'Menopause: Mind the Gap'. I included this because I want my readers to be equipped with the information and statistics they need to make the case for support in the workplace.

How to use this book

It is your choice how you use this book. You can read it all to get a complete picture of menopause, or dip in and out of it if you just want to read the bits that relate to something you are currently experiencing or concerned about.

Chapter 1 provides you with some definitions and information that will be useful to you if you want to discuss your symptoms with your doctor or other health professionals.

Chapters 2-8 relate to the most common menopausal symptoms. Each chapter includes information, techniques and comments from real women about their experiences.

In Chapter 9 I have brought together my 10 Top Tips to control menopause symptoms.

Chapter 10 provides the background to why menopause is a workplace issue.

In the Resources section I have included a chart of menopausal symptoms that you can use to record your experiences for your own information or to share with your doctor or other medical professional if you are seeking advice. There are also links to the bonus journals relating to specific symptoms so that you can keep track of any changes resulting from actions you are taking.

I have included some useful book titles and websites if you are interested in further reading on the subject.

Let me reassure you that you are not alone in what you are experiencing. Millions of women have walked this path and millions are on it with you. Let's support each other and do this together.

CHAPTER 1

WHAT IS THE MENOPAUSE?

The term menopause is often used to refer generally to the years of women's lives either side of their last menstrual period. It is sometimes called 'the change' or 'time of life'. More technically correct terms are defined below.

Menopause can occur as early as 40 or not until 55 but the average age in the UK is 52 and 51 in the USA. However, you can also start to experience menopausal symptoms earlier as you enter into the phase known as 'perimenopause'.

Menopause that occurs before the age of 40 is known medically as premature ovarian failure (POF) or primary ovarian insufficiency (POI). This occurs in 1 to 4 per cent of women. Early menopause can be precipitated by illnesses and medical interventions including radiotherapy and hysterectomy, but in up to 70 per cent of cases there is no obvious medical reason. In these cases it is advisable to seek medical investigation.

Men experience some menopausal-type symptoms as their hormone levels change in mid-life. This period is known as 'andropause'. Symptoms can include body shape changes, weight gain, hot flushes and mood swings.

Some Definitions

Various terms are used in connection with menopause and some of them can be a bit confusing. It is useful to understand what is generally meant by these terms, particularly if you want to talk to health professionals

Climacteric – the ongoing changes and symptoms that occur during the transition period when ovarian and hormonal production decline. This stage may last 15-20 years between the ages of 40 and 60. It can be compared to the years of puberty and adolescence.

Premature menopause, premature ovarian failure or primary ovarian insufficiency – menopause that occurs before the age of 40. May have an identified medical reason or no known reason. If your periods stop before age 40 you should seek medical advice.

Pre-menopause – the early years of the transition period when menopause symptoms may be experienced. Generally, this stage starts after the age of 40 and goes on until menstrual periods cease.

Perimenopause – this is the stage either side of your last menstrual period when you notice most physical changes and symptoms, and when periods may become more or less frequent before stopping completely.

Menopause – one year after your last menstrual period.

Post-menopause – the years after your last period up to the end of your life. It overlaps with the perimenopause.

Andropause – the male menopause. Men produce less testosterone after the age of 40. This can lead to fewer and harder to sustain erections, hot flushes, lethargy, mood swings, irritability and decreased sexual desire.

In this book I will mainly be talking about perimenopause.

Hormones related to reproduction and menopause

As women come towards the end of the reproductive stage of their lives, the supply of eggs reduces and the levels of hormones associated with reproduction begin to decline. This results in the end of menstruation and physical changes to the body.

The reproductive hormones involved are:

Oestrogen – is most commonly thought of as the 'female hormone' although men also produce it. Women produce three forms of oestrogen; oestradiol, oestrone, and oestriol. Oestrogen helps to develop our sexual characteristics and also supports many bodily processes.

Progesterone – is the key hormone in pregnancy. It helps to maintain pregnancy and prevents further fertilisation. It is the hormone that triggers the menstrual bleed.

Follicle Stimulating Hormone (FSH) – is a hormone that stimulates the ovaries to produce eggs. High levels of FSH may indicate an impending menopause.

Testosterone – small amounts of testosterone are produced by women in the ovaries and adrenal glands. Not much is known about the role of testosterone in women, but scientists believe it helps to maintain muscle and bone strength and contributes to confidence, sex drive, and libido.

What will my menopause be like?

There are a number of factors that affect the nature of the menopausal symptoms women experience.

- Genetics. One indication of your possible experience is what happened to your mother and your close female relatives during their menopause. Their experiences can give you a clue to the timing and symptoms you might expect. Remember, you only share 50% of your DNA with your mother so your experience may not be the same.

- Nutrition. The diet you have had during your lifetime is likely to be very different to the diet your mother and female relatives of her age experienced. The quantity and quality of your nutrition will influence the nature of your perimenopause.

- Lifestyle. There are a number of lifestyle factors that have been shown to affect menopausal symptoms including stress, exercise, smoking, and drinking alcohol. More controversially, studies in the UK and Australia have shown that women with higher education levels and social class were less likely to experience vasomotor symptoms (eg hot flashes and night sweats) than other women (UQ News, 2012).

- Mindset. Your mindset at menopause, whether negative or positive, will impact on your menopause symptoms.

- Health. Your underlying health may affect the nature and intensity of your menopause symptoms, particularly if you are taking medication or undergoing treatment.

All of this means that you do not have to be a victim of your genes. The decisions you take all through your life about your diet, exercise, and lifestyle will have an equally significant effect on your experience of menopause and your health in later life. It's never too early to plan for a healthy menopause, and it is never too late to have a healthy lifestyle.

How will you know if you are in the perimenopause stage?

While many women may have little or no doubt when they start going through the stages of menopause, others have only minimal discomfort and can be unsure about what they are experiencing. This may be a particular issue if the symptoms start to occur before age 40.

If you are experiencing regular menopause symptoms, such as changes to menstrual periods, hot flashes, night sweats, and/or vaginal dryness, you may want to have a test to confirm the cause.

You can purchase a home-test kit to measure your level of FSH. A positive test indicates that you may be in a stage of menopause.

Alternatively, you can seek advice from your medical practitioner who may carry out an FSH or other tests.

There is a Menopause Symptoms Record in the Resources section of this book. You can use it to make a note of the frequency and intensity of any symptoms that you are experiencing. This will be useful information if you decide to seek medical advice. You can also download and print off an extended version of this record at www.hotwomencoolsolutions.com

HRT or not?

Hormone Replacement Therapy (HRT), also referred to as Hormone Therapy, has been available since the 1930s. The earliest prescription drug for oestrogen was called Premarin which was an oral medication made from the urine of pregnant horses. This was followed by a synthetic form of progesterone called Prempro. HRT medications contain various combinations of oestrogen and progestin.

Initially, it was thought to be safe for women to start taking HRT at the onset of menopausal symptoms and to stay on it for the rest of their lives. Following the report of the Women's Health Initiative in 2002 it was recommended that women only stay on HRT for the short term (such as 5 years) due to the potential health risks such as increased risk of heart attacks, blood clots, and breast cancer.

The WHI Report had a chilling effect on the prescription and demand for HRT. In recent years, more research has been carried out into the risks and benefits of HRT. It is essential for women considering taking HRT to discuss the health implications with their doctor or other medical professional.

It is important to remember that when you stop taking HRT you may experience menopause symptoms no matter what age you are.

Most women seek HRT to control hot flushes and night sweats but some also consider taking it because they think that it will keep their hair and skin looking good, and also give them more energy and a better sex drive. Research published in 2003 (NEJM, 2003) concluded that *"In this trial in postmenopausal women, oestrogen plus progestin did not have a clinically meaningful effect on health-related quality of life".*

There is a large range of HRT products available which are manufactured from an array of ingredients. It can be administered in a variety of forms:

- Implants. A pellet containing a six month supply of oestrogen is inserted under the skin of the lower abdomen. The hormones are delivered directly into the bloodstream, and that means that the dose can be lower. The disadvantage is that it can be difficult to remove the implant if you decide to stop HRT.

- Tablets. This is the most common way of taking HRT where oestrogen is taken every day and progestogen is taken from day 15 to day 25 of the cycle. With this combination you continue to have menstrual bleeds. There is also a no-bleed option called Livial. It is recommended that this is only prescribed when you have had one complete year free of periods.

- Skin patches. Skin patches deliver hormones directly to the bloodstream through the skin and, as with the implants, this means that the required dose is lower, reducing side effects. They are worn on the hip, upper thigh or lower abdomen. Patches are available as oestrogen only or as combined oestrogen and progestogen. They are applied once or twice a week depending on the brand. The disadvantages are that dose adjustments are difficult and some women develop a skin reaction to the patch

- Vaginal rings, pessaries and creams. Preparations containing oestrogen to be applied directly to the vagina can be prescribed to ease symptoms such as vaginal dryness, itching, burning or discharge. The advantage is that the hormone is delivered directly to the oestrogen depleted area. Most preparations are only licensed for use for 3-6 months of continuous use.

- Gels and creams. Oestrogen gels and creams rubbed on to the skin are absorbed easily and enter into the circulatory system. They are applied to a specific are of the body every day using the right and left hand side of the body on alternate days. They are generally rapid drying which eliminates problems of them rubbing off or being transferred to another person.

Like all medications, HRT can have unpleasant side-effects including depression, skin rashes, hair loss, vomiting bloating and cystitis-like syndrome. It can increase health risks for some women particularly those who smoke, have high blood pressure, benign breast disease, endometriosis, pancreatitis, epilepsy, or migraines.

If the first formulation of HRT that you are prescribed does not deal with your symptoms, be prepared to go back to your medical practitioner or consultant to ask for a review.

Bio-Identical Hormone Therapy (BIHT)

Bio-identical hormones have been prescribed in America for many years and are now available in the UK. They have structures identical to human hormones and are mostly derived from plant sources including soy or Mexican yam root. Although they are considered to be 'more natural' than other HRT products, the plant compounds undergo synthetic processing to obtain the hormones used.

Common components of compounded bio-identical hormone formulations include estrone, estriol, testosterone, and micronized progesterone. There are bio-identical hormone products which are manufactured by big pharmaceutical companies, for example Crinone and Utrogest. These products undergo trials and testing in order to be approved by national health organisations such as the US Food and Drug Administration (FDA), the UK Medicines and Healthcare products Regulatory Authority (MHRA), and the Australian Therapeutic Goods Administration (TGA).

Other BIHT products are produced by compounding pharmacies according to the individual formulation of the prescribing practitioner. Practitioners prescribe a compound of hormones tailored to the needs of the individual, often based on the results of saliva and blood tests.

As with HRT, BIHT can take a variety of forms including tablets and creams to suit different symptoms. Practitioners will normally aim to treat with the lowest dose for the shortest period of time.

It is possible to purchase bio-identical hormones over the internet but it is inadvisable to self-medicate. These are drugs and they carry risks and the chance of side effects. Always discuss the options with your doctor or a consultant.

Self-Advocacy

If you are experiencing moderate or severe menopausal symptoms you may be considering some form of hormone therapy. It is debatable whether BIHT is any more natural or lower risk than HRT. All forms of HRT have a long list of contraindications and possible side effects.

The important thing in making this decision is to be well informed about the benefits and the risks before you discuss the options with your doctor. Good communication between the doctor and the patient is the key to effective treatment.

There are some references for further reading in the Resources section at the end of this book.

'I was lucky enough to have an easy menopause. Although my periods started to become irregular when I was only 37, it was only by a few days and not a problem. I can't remember when I first experienced hot flushes. The main thing I remember is being too busy to take much notice of them. But I'm realistic enough to know that means they weren't very bad. I've certainly seen women suffer much, much more. I just took off a layer or two of clothes or stood outside until it passed.' Teresa

"I was 43 when I had a hot flash and I thought 'that's enough of that!' My bone density was low anyway and an early menopause could have led to osteoporosis. I went to see the doctor and was put on HRT. I stayed on it for 10 years and then life got a bit hectic and I didn't bother going back to the doctor to renew my prescription. I have not had any menopause symptoms since so I consider myself quite lucky." Mary

"I have recently had a full hysterectomy to remove large fibroids which were causing very heavy periods. It was recommended I take HRT to avoid immediate menopause symptoms which could be caused by the ovaries being removed during surgery. I use an oestrogen only gel. It is very easy - I simply rub it into my thigh once a day. My surgeon believes HRT provides many long term health benefits and I should stay on my current dose until age 65. At this age I can then go on to half my current dose but continue taking it. My understanding is the thinking around previous health worries thought to be associated with taking HRT is changing (eg increased risk of breast cancer). The gel is also considered to be better as the oestrogen is absorbed via the skin directly into the bloodstream.

It's now 7 weeks since the operation and I'm beginning to feel really well. I hadn't noticed any menopause symptoms before the operation

and feel fortunate that I do not need to go through a potentially uncomfortable time. I love going long distance walking and can now go without worrying about where to change a tampon!" Karen

"I started taking HRT 20 years ago. Back then we didn't know anything about the health risks associated with taking HRT over many years. I also didn't realise that if I stopped taking HRT I would have to go through the menopause. I am 70 now and I don't want to start having menopause symptoms so I suppose I will just keep taking the tablets." Ellen

"I was diagnosed with early menopause on my thirty-sixth birthday when my son was 18 months old.

I was recommended to take HRT and I did a lot of research into the risks and benefits. I realised it came with a lot of health warnings. I read all the information about how HRT can increase the risk of breast cancer and other health issues, and it was really quite conflicting information. I couldn't find anything specific about early menopause.

I spoke to my consultant, and he said, 'Do you want to be running around in the park with your son and you fall and break your leg?' He was letting me know that because I was young, without HRT I could lose bone density. I decided to go ahead and take HRT. I was prescribed a combined pill but after three months they weren't having much effect. After two further changes to my prescription HRT started to work for me, it really helped me get back to normal.

I also made changes to my diet and exercise which made an enormous difference. I feel like I am 99% back to normal now." Lesley

Chapter 2

HOW CAN I STAY COOL AND SLEEP BETTER?

Hot flashes are one of the most common symptoms that send women to see their doctors when they are going through the perimenopause. About 60% of women experience hot flashes and/or night sweats and of those, 70% experience them for a year, and 30% for about 5 years (Foxcroft, 2009). So, it is surprising that so little is known about what causes them and what is going on inside the body when a woman has one.

Researcher and Author, Lisa Mosconi, suggests that hot flashes are the result of a lack of oestrogen in the brain. The hypothalmus regulates body temperature. "When oestrogen doesn't activate the hypothalamus correctly, the brain cannot regulate body temperature correctly. So those hot flashes that women get, that's the hypothalamus." (Lisa Mosconi, 2019)

The intensity and duration of hot flashes varies from woman to woman. During a hot flash the blood vessels dilate, increasing the flow of blood to the skin, most noticeably to the face, neck and chest but also in the back. A rise in temperature is accompanied by sensations of heat, sometimes overwhelming, followed by sweating and cooling down. Some women also experience increased heart rate, dizziness, faintness, and nausea. A hot flash generally lasts between 3 and 5 minutes

Not every woman who has hot flashes also has night sweats, but if they have hot flushes at night, they can wake up hot and drenched in sweat. Night sweats may occur several times a night and can result in interrupted sleep. It is important to note that night sweats can be related to non-menopausal issues such as stress and you should consult your doctor if you are unsure of the cause.

The implications of hot flashes have been subject to many research projects but the results are not consistent. One study has shown that women who suffer from hot flashes and night sweats may be at lower risk for cardiovascular disease and stroke. *"While they are certainly bothersome, hot flashes may not be all bad,"* according to Northwestern Medicine endocrinologist Emily Szmuilowicz, MD, who is lead author of the study. *"Our research found that despite previous reports suggesting that menopause symptoms were associated with increased levels of risk markers for heart disease, such as blood pressure and cholesterol, the actual outcomes tell a different story."*

Other studies suggest that the parasympathetic nervous system works less well during hot flashes (Goodwin, J. 2012). Although this effect is transient, as the parasympathetic nervous system regulates the body at rest, more research is being done in this area.

Several studies have concluded that women who lose weight could experience fewer menopausal symptoms including hot flashes. A study by the journal 'Menopause' found that women who followed a low-fat, high fruit, vegetable and fibre diet lost weight and had significantly reduced hot flashes and night sweats. One reason for this could be that body fat can prevent heat loss because it acts as insulation. For more advice on weight and diet see Chapter 3 How do I control my weight?

Sleep

As already mentioned, hot flushes and night sweats can lead to poor or disrupted sleep. During a good night's sleep, you have balanced periods of slow-wave sleep, where your body carries out physical housekeeping, and rapid eye movement sleep (REM) where your brain processes memories from the day.

Poor sleep is characterised by longer periods of REM and shorter slow-wave sleep. This type of pattern can lead to you feeling tired when you wake up in the morning because your body has not had sufficient rest

Good sleep is important because it:

● Rejuvenates the body

● Enhances health:

- ○ Lowers risk of heart problems

- ○ May prevent cancer

- ○ Reduces stress

- ○ Reduces inflammation

- ○ May help to control weight

- Aids memory

- Energises

- Lifts mood

People vary in how much sleep they need. Some people believe that they are sleep deprived if they are not getting eight hours sleep a night, or as much sleep as they used to when they were younger. However, not everyone needs eight hours sleep.

If you function well during the day, you are probably getting enough sleep. In this case, you can stop lying in bed worrying about not getting enough sleep.

What you can do to improve sleep

Over time, hot flashes get milder and less frequent and, for most women, they eventually disappear altogether. If they are particularly severe and debilitating, you may want to consider medical treatment such as HRT or sleep medication. Otherwise, there are some diet and lifestyle changes that you can make that may assist.

Before you start to make any changes, it is helpful to identify any patterns of good or poor sleep by keeping a sleep journal for a week. You can download a Sleep Journal template at www.hotwomencoolsolutions.com

Diet

There are changes that you can make to your diet that will help you to balance your hormones:

- Eliminate triggers from your diet - you can identify these from your Journal. Common triggers include sugar, caffeine, chocolate, alcohol, and spicy foods

- Make sure you drink enough to stay well hydrated – preferably water or cool drinks

- Include phytoestrogens* in your diet to balance your hormones, for example:

  o Isoflavines – soya, chickpeas, lentils and kidney beans

  o Lignans – flaxseeds (linseeds) sesame seeds, sunflower seeds, brown rice, oats, broccoli and carrots

  o Coumestans – found in sprouted mung beans and alfalfa beans

- Eat more omega 3 fatty acids – found in sardines, salmon, mackerel and flaxseeds (linseeds).

*These foods are often not recommended for women who have been treated for breast cancer. Check with your oncologist.

For best effect eat organic, unprocessed foods whenever possible.

Sleep medication

In the UK, more than 10 million prescriptions are given for sleeping pills every year. Medication offers only short term relief because sleeping tablets treat the symptoms of poor sleep and not the causes. Medical practitioners are advised to prescribe drugs only after considering non-drug therapies

If you are thinking of taking sleeping tablets or are already taking them, there are some things you might want to consider. Not all sleeping pills are the same. Each class of sleep aid works a bit differently, and side effects vary.

It's important to ask key questions before choosing your sleep medicine.

- o How long does it take for the sleeping pill to take effect?

- o How long do the effects last?

- o What is the risk of becoming dependent on the sleeping medication, physically or psychologically?

There are three categories of prescription drugs your doctor may recommend.

1. Benzodiazepine hypnotics can be highly effective. Yet, for some people they can be too heavily sedating making them feel groggy and exhausted the next day. They also have a propensity to cause physical dependency. Drug names include Temazepam, Ativan, Xanax, and Halcion.

2. Non-Benzodiazepines like Ambien, Lunesta and Sonata are a newer class of sleep medicine, which are less likely to cause addiction. People also report feeling more refreshed when they awaken after taking this type of medication.

3. Antidepressants such as Aventyl, Desyrel, and Paxil are sometimes prescribed to help people sleep because these medications have a sedating effect.

Non-prescription medicines

There are many over the counter remedies available at a pharmacy. The common ingredient in all these pills is an antihistamine, which causes drowsiness. So whatever you choose you are essentially getting the same type of medicine.

Always check with your doctor before taking over-the-counter sleep medication. Even commonly available sleeping pills can cause side effects and interact with other medication you are taking. So, exercise caution and take only as directed by your doctor.

Complementary therapies

There is a range of complementary therapies that you can you to help to alleviate sleep problems.

Herbal Remedies. There is some evidence that the herb valerian is effective for insomnia. Passionflower, hops, lavender, lemon balm, and Jamaica dogwood are also traditionally used to help with sleep, but their benefits have not been proven in medical trials. If you are taking any other medication, check with your doctor or pharmacist before taking any herbal remedies.

Homeopathic remedies. Homeopaths do not usually prescribe remedies for individual symptoms, instead the remedy is to treat the whole person. Some common remedies for sleep disorders include:

- Arnica – for overwork and when the bed feels hard and uncomfortable

- Aconite – for acute insomnia caused by shock, fright, bad news or grief

- Kali phos – night terrors exhausted by stress or overwork

- Lachesis – night sweats

- Pulsatilla – early waking with over-active mind

- Sepia – difficulty falling asleep Night sweats

Aromatherapy: A few drop of some essential oils added to a warm bath before bed can help to ease sleep problems. Lavender oil is anti-inflammatory and has a mildly sedative effect. Chamomile and ylang-ylang also appear to improve sleep.

Warning: some people may experience skin irritation when using essential oils. Essential oils should never be applied directly to the skin.

Lifestyle changes

Very minor changes in core body temperature can be a trigger for hot flashes in some women. You can avoid over-heating by:

- Using a fan at work and at home

- Wearing layered clothing, preferably in natural fibres, so that you can remove and replace layers as required

- Keeping your bedroom cool and well-ventilated

- Sleeping under a light duvet or loosely woven blanket. If you are sleeping with a partner you could consider separate duvets or covers.

- Exercising regularly in the morning to stay healthy and allow your rate of metabolism to slow before bedtime

If you are experiencing poor or interrupted sleep, check the quality of your bedroom environment. Your bedroom should be a sleep haven. Most people sleep better in a room that is dark, cool and quiet. Remove the TV, computers, and smart phones from the bedroom so that there are no distractions from sleep. Also, consider whether you need to buy a more comfortable mattress or different pillows.

Your Bonus

You can download a relaxation/hypnotic recording to aid better sleep at www.hotwomencoolsolutions.com

"Hot flushes have not been easy at times to handle, especially the night sweats. My nights are disturbed by the fluctuating temperature and I guess that it is easier that I live on my own so that I do not disturb a partner.

I have had the experience of waking with sweat running down my chest which is uncomfortable and could be embarrassing if I was sleeping with somebody. When I have been with other people and have had a hot flush sometimes the people that I have been with thought that it was funny. That has made me feel uncomfortable."
Sally

"I have had hot flushes for about six years. Stress and uncomfortable situations can bring on a flush. I sometimes feel like I'm going to have a heart attack. At one time I was having over 50 flushes a day. I perspire right down my nose. I can reduce mine now using my internal control panel. It makes me feel more in control.

I sleep on silk sheets. The coolness of them cools down my pulse points at night and reduces my night sweats." Rose

"The hot flushes started at about age 50 and they got worse and worse. I perspired so much I had to leave my job in a jeweller's because I was leaving wet hand prints on the counter! Physical heat, hot drinks, spicy foods, and stress make me flush more.

I can't stop them but I can control them now using visualisation. I visualise standing in wellington boots in water or standing in the snow. That cools me down fast. I feel like I can get it under control." Martha

"I had started to experience regular hot flashes and night sweats just before I went on holiday to Japan. During the two weeks I was there I ate a traditional Japanese diet with lots of fish, soy products, vegetables, and green tea. The hot flashes stopped straight away and only came back when I got back home!" Amelia

COOL SOLUTIONS

Cooling breath

There is a yoga breathing technique known as 'Shitali' that is used to cool down the body. Do not use this technique if you have a respiratory or heart condition.

1. Stick your tongue out of your mouth as far as possible without straining.

2. Roll the sides of the tongue inwards so that it forms a circular shape.

3. Inhale through the mouth, drawing the air over the tongue.

4. Pull your tongue back inside your mouth and exhale through your nose.

Visualisation

Visualisation is the process of forming mental images. To make images in your mind you can use memories or construct an image or use a combination of both. For example, if I ask you to imagine a Caribbean beach you could use a memory if you have been there, or you could construct an image from pictures that you have seen, or descriptions that you've heard.

All emotions begin with a thought and the pictures and conversation we have in our minds in relation to that thought. Being able to visualise an outcome we want can stimulate and mobilise the activity of the nervous system to achieve that outcome. In other words, if you want something good to happen, start by creating a picture in your mind of what that good thing would look like.

You might have already experienced the effect of visualisation. Have you ever been watching a film or TV programme about somewhere cold or icy like the Arctic or Everest, and as you watched it did you start to feel colder? This is because your brain is imagining you being in that place and generates those physical sensations of coldness.

Visualisation is used for a number of purposes including improving sports performance, problem solving, innovation, therapy, and healing. Research has shown that being able to visualise cool images helps to reduce the experience of hot flashes, particularly if this is included within hypnosis. A study by Baylor's College of Arts and Sciences showed that hot flushes could be reduced by up to 68% in women who visualised cool places such as mountains, waterfalls, and snow.

Most people are all able to visualise although some find it easier than others. If you don't find it easy you may need to practice, starting with some familiar images for example:

- Picture your front door.

- Picture your car

- Picture an apple

- Picture a loved one's face

Everyone* is different in how they picture things and what makes the emotions associated with those images stronger or weaker. Before you start using the visualisations below try the following exercise so that you know what makes your images particularly effective.

1. Think of a time when you felt calm and relaxed and allow an image of that situation to form in your mind. On a scale of 1 to 10, notice how strong that feeling is as you look at that image.

2. Move that image away from you and make it smaller. How strong is the feeling now?

3. Move the image towards you and make it bigger. How strong is that feeling now?

4. Repeat this process making the picture black and white and then colour, flat and 3D, moving and still. Notice what happens to that feeling of calm and relaxation. Does it get stronger or weaker?

*If you find visualisation too difficult, do this exercise using whatever sense works best for you, for example imagine the calm feelings in your body, or calm, relaxing sounds. Make those feelings or sounds stronger in whatever way is right for you to really experience it.

When you first start using this technique, you might want to have an actual image of somewhere or something really cold in front of you that you can look at to trigger the feelings of coolness.

Visualisation is most effective if you do it regularly. You could start by doing it for 1 minute, 3 times a day and work up to doing it for 10 minutes three times a day. The more regularly you do it, the easier it will become to construct the image and feel the cooling physical effect when you need it.

There are some examples below but if you are used to visualising, you may want to construct some cool images of your own.

1. Cool Visualisations

1. Walking in the rain. Picture yourself looking out of your window watching it raining outside. Cool, Spring rain. Now, picture yourself going to the door and stepping outside, feeling the rain gently falling on your head, running down your hair and face, cool and refreshing. And as you continue

to walk out in the shower, a gentle breeze is blowing. You can feel the coolness all over your body, spreading down from your head, though your shoulders, your chest, down though your stomach all the way down to your feet. Carry on imagining being outside in the rain for as long you want to and really enjoy that cool feeling.

2. Put out the furnace. Imagine a furnace inside you that is spreading heat all through your body. The furnace is glowing red, you can see flames inside and there are sparks flying out of the top. Now, imagine taking a hose and starting to spray water all over the furnace. See the water cooling off the furnace, the sparks die away, and the flames are put out. The colour gradually fades away as the furnace cools down and the water continues to flow all over it from the top to the bottom.

2. Control Panel

This technique also uses visualisation

Your Temperature Control Panel

Step 1 Visualise a central control room in your head. It has all the dials and indicators that control the balance of the body.

Step 2 Find the control panel for your body temperature. Put a scale on the control from 1 to 10, where 1 is cold, 5 is comfortable, and 10 is very hot. Colour the numbers from 1 to 3 white, 4 to 7 is blue, and the numbers 8,9 and 10 red.

Step 3 Notice where your body temperature is on that scale at the moment. See what number the indicator is pointing at.

Step 4 Move the indicator on your scale up towards 10. As you do that, notice how the temperature in your body changes.

Step 5 Now move the indicator on your scale down towards 1, and notice again how the temperature in your body changes.

Once you can easily access your temperature control, practice moving it up and down so that whenever you start to feel too warm you can just adjust the control to level that's comfortable for you.

3. Self-hypnosis

Self-hypnosis is a useful technique for getting back to sleep during the night but you could also use it to relax and de-stress during the day.

1. Sit or lie down comfortably in a quiet room where you know you will not be disturbed for at least 15 minutes. Make any adjustments to be completely comfortable.

2. Close your eyes and focus on your breathing, without trying to change it. Notice your thoughts and let them just slip away.

3. Send your attention around your body noticing any sensations or aches and pains without judging them or putting any meaning to them.

4. Start letting go of any tension in your body. Beginning at your toes, tense them, and then relax them. Flex your feet and relax them. Move up your body tensing and relaxing your muscles.

5. When your attention gets to your head, clench and relax your jaw. Imagine your cheeks and then the top of your head being gently massaged.

6. Continue to breathe slowly and deeply. Recognise how relaxed you are feeling. You may feel like you are floating or sinking. You can use that feeling and send yourself a positive message by repeating an affirmation to yourself for example 'I am cool and comfortable', or 'I am drifting off into deep and refreshing sleep', or 'I am successful and positive'. Repeat your statement as many times as seems appropriate.

7. If you are going through this process at night, you can let yourself drift off to sleep. If you are relaxing during the day, you can let your consciousness return to the room, noticing your surroundings and saying out loud 'Wide Awake' or 'Back in the room'.

If you find this technique difficult, you could buy a pre-recorded hypnosis track or download a relaxation app. If you can, listen to a sample before you buy so that you know whether the voice in the recording is right for you. Some voices sound like finger nails on a blackboard!

Chapter 3

HOW DO I CONTROL MY WEIGHT?

Body changes

Just as during puberty, hormonal changes during perimenopause bring about changes to your weight and body shape. At this stage of your life, your metabolism will be slowing down and you may be naturally losing muscle which helps you to burn off fat.

During this phase of your life, your ovaries produce less oestrogen and your body tries to compensate by manufacturing oestrogen elsewhere to protect your body against osteoporosis. The fat around the middle of your body is one of the sites where oestrogen is produced and stored. So, a little bit of weight gain around your waist is not your body turning against you – it's trying to support you!

Strategies that you have used in the past to lose weight may not work as well now. Calorie controlled diets are not the answer. Diets make your body think that you are being starved and as soon as you eat 'normally' again, it will replenish the fat stores in case there is a famine again! A better approach is about a long-term, different relationship to food.

It is useful to keep a Food Journal to help you to identify any patterns of how, when and what you eat. You can download a journal at www.hotwomencoolsolutions.com

Apples v Pears

The first sign of the start of perimenopause for some women may be gaining weight around the waist and changing to an 'apple' shape. Alternatively, you may put weight on around your hips and thighs giving rise to the 'pear' shape.

As explained above, a small amount of weight gain around your middle is okay. However, excessive fat in that area can be a sign of stress and can be dangerous for your health and particularly your risk of breast cancer (Glenville, 2006)

The time to take action is if your waist to hip ratio exceeds 0.8. To calculate this, measure your waist and hips and then divide your waist by your hip measurement. If your ratio is higher than 0.8 it can increase your risk of a range of conditions including cancer, high blood pressure and stroke.

The 'Mindful Eating' advice below applies to 'Apples' and 'Pears'. For more advice on losing weight around your waist see 'Fat Around the Middle' by Marilyn Glenville.

Underweight

This is not about being naturally slim or thin, this is about your weight being too low to support your health and wellbeing. Being underweight is an issue at any stage of a woman's life. When you are younger if you are underweight, it can affect your periods and your fertility. During perimenopause it can increase your risk of osteoporosis.

If you are generally eating well and you are losing weight you should seek advice from your doctor. It can be a sign of other health issues such as an overactive thyroid or coeliac disease.

Mindful Eating

If you want to lose weight or maintain a healthy weight, the first step is to understand the difference between physical and emotional hunger and only eat when you are physically hungry.

Physical hunger comes on slowly. You might gradually feel loss of energy, loss of concentration, irritable, lightheaded, empty, hunger pangs in stomach and, finally, must eat now! If you eat something when you are physically hungry, the hunger indicators will gradually fade away.

Emotional hunger comes on suddenly. You might start to salivate because you saw or smelt food, get the oral urge to chew, or search through the cupboards to find something to satisfy a craving or feel sadness, anger or frustration. If you eat when you are emotionally hungry, you are likely to feel unsatisfied, and possibly even sick.

If you start to eat before you are physically hungry you won't know when to stop eating. Also, if you do not eat when you start to feel hungry you are more likely to start to crave carbohydrates. When you are starving hungry, a salad doesn't look appealing whereas a baguette or a sticky bun looks just right. Therefore, being aware of your current level of hunger is important (see 'Cool Solutions' below).

The signals for thirst and hunger are very similar so, if you start to feel hungry, have a drink of water and then wait for ten minutes to feel if the hunger signal is still there. If it is, go ahead and eat.

The second step to losing or maintaining weight is to stop eating when you are satisfied. Do not wait for the 'full' or 'stuffed' signal as you will have eaten too much. There are two hormones that play an important role in regulating appetite and weight, ghrelin and leptin.

Ghrelin is produced by the stomach and it sends the message that you need to eat. Ghrelin levels fall when the food you eat arrives at your intestines. If you go on an extreme diet, more ghrelin gets secreted and your ability to burn calories starts to diminish.

Leptin is a hormone secreted by fat cells which regulates appetite and metabolism. Levels of leptin rise as we eat so that the appetite is suppressed. It also promotes calorie burning.

The levels of leptin and ghrelin can also be affected by your sleep patterns. Studies have found that people who regularly slept for just 5 hours a night had 15% more ghrelin in their system, leading to feelings of hunger. They also had significantly less leptin to suppress the appetite. In light of this research, it is important to sort out any sleep issues before you try to lose weight (see Chapter 2: How can I keep cool and sleep better?)

The secret to recognising these signals and having time to react to them is to eat mindfully, that is:

- Sit down when you eat—even if it's only a snack.

- Take time to enjoy your food - look at, smell and taste the food

- Slow down - put the knife and fork down between mouthfuls

- Chew your food completely

- Drink before you eat - don't drink while you are eating

- Concentrate on eating - don't do anything but eat ie no TV, radio or reading

- Eat three meals a day – it is easier to keep track of your food intake if you eat regular meals rather than 'grazing'

Right Foods

There is plenty of expert diet and nutrition advice available but the frustrating thing is that so much of it is contradictory. We accept the Government's advice about having 5 portions of fruit and vegetables a day, but other countries recommend 7 portions and some as many as 9 portions!

You can gain weight on any food and you can lose weight on any food so, eat things that you enjoy, but only eat between the levels of hunger and satisfaction. If you find it hard to leave food on the plate at the end of a meal, and many people do, take care with your portion size. Your body only wants about a fist size portion of food at any one feeding. By tuning into the signals coming from your stomach what you want to eat and what your body most wants to eat will gradually become the same.

By eating proteins, such as lean meats and nuts, the level of ghrelin in your system stays lower and you feel fuller longer. If you eat simple sugars and carbohydrates the level of ghrelin will spike and you will feel hungry again quickly.

There are also lots of food myths to be aware of. For example, there is the myth that fat free food is calorie free. In fact 'Low fat' and 'Fat Free' foods are often higher in sugars and chemicals to add back flavour. Therefore, they can be more fattening and less nutritious than regular food. It is always a good idea to check the labels on food before you buy.

If you are eating out at a fast-food restaurant many of them offer a 'healthy option', but beware. A 2005 report found that 5 out of 8 salads sold by McDonalds, Burger King, KFC and Pizza Hut had high salt or fat content. For example, a Big Mac had 540 calories and 1040 mg of salt; a premium southwest salad with crispy chicken and dressing had 530 calories and 1,260 mg of salt.

The lesson from all this is that it is better to eat simple, unprocessed foods whenever possible so that you know exactly what you are eating.

Some general food guidelines:

- Start the day with breakfast—people who do find it easier to lose weight. Eating protein at breakfast will keep you feeling fuller for longer

- Keep your diet healthy, balanced and satisfying

- Soup stays longer in the stomach and delays hunger pangs

- Eat vegetables that grow above ground – they store less sugar

- Watch your portion size - reducing the size of your plate will reduce your food intake

- Don't skip meals. If you let yourself get too hungry you will want to eat carbohydrates

Eating out can be a real challenge when you are establishing new eating habits and trying to lose weight. When you are eating socially what's important isn't the food – it's the company. The problem is that when you are chatting with your friends you can lose track of what you are eating and how you are eating it. A few alcoholic drinks not only add calories they also make you less aware of the amount of food you are consuming.

Whether you are eating in a restaurant or at a dinner party keep to the same guidelines for mindful eating, that is: eat slowly, and stop eating as soon as you are satisfied. Some more tips:

- Push the bread basket away and resist the temptation to eat before your meal starts by sipping water and chatting to your companions. If the bread rolls are served by a waiter just smile and say "Not for me, thank you".

• Don't over-order or overload your plate. You may be able to order two starters instead of a starter and a main course.

• You don't have to eat everything on your plate. If it really upsets you to leave food on your plate in a restaurant ask for a doggie bag. At dinner parties just say "That was great, I'm really full."

• Ask for sauce or gravy on the side so that you can have a smaller amount.

• Trade potatoes for an extra vegetable that you enjoy

• If you want a dessert, share one with a friend.

Alcohol can be an issue if you are experiencing hot flushes. There is no reason why you can't enjoy a drink (unless otherwise advised by your doctor), so long as you drink in moderation and make sensible choices. Weight for weight, alcohol contains more calories than sugar, so even moderate drinking can lead to weight gain.When days don't go to plan don't give up. While you are establishing new eating habits and a new relationship to food there will be days when it is difficult. But if you keep going back to the guidelines they will just become how you normally eat and you won't have to think about them anymore. This is not an 'all or nothing' approach.

Do not check your weight every day. While you are peri-menopausal, your weight will continue to fluctuate with your hormone levels. If you weigh-in every day there will be days when it goes up and that can be a bit disheartening. Once a fortnight is enough, once a month is even better.

Food Supplements

If you want to lose weight there are supplements that claim to help your body burn off excess fat and reduce stress hormones. These weight-related supplements typically contain one or more of the following:

> Chromium – to control insulin levels
>
> B vitamins – for glucose metabolism and to balance blood sugar
>
> Magnesium – for the calming effect on the body
>
> Zinc – to aid the production of hormones, including leptin
>
> Vitamin C – to regulate blood sugar
>
> Omega 3 fats – to help burn off fat

There has been quite a lot written about the links between vitamin D and obesity, and whether weight loss influences the levels of vitamin D available in the blood. Vitamin D is important for bone health and may have a protective role against heart disease and cancer. The evidence relating to the link with weight loss is inconclusive and the general advice is to take vitamin D as part of a multi-vitamin supplement (Saunders, T. 2011).

All supplements should be used as directed and in conjunction with the healthier approach to eating outlined above. There is more information about food supplements in the Resources section.

Exercise

When you are trying to lose or maintain weight you are often given the 'eat less, exercise more' or the 'calories in, calories burnt' message, but the science behind this is a lot less straightforward than it seems (Harcombe, 2011).

What is indisputable is that exercise is good for your mental and physical wellbeing. Exercise will speed up your metabolic rate which will help to burn off calories. This does not mean that you need to sign up for the gym. There are plenty of additional activities and exercises that you can do at home (see Chapter 5 What can I do to stay fit and healthy?).

Be aware that if you do additional exercise you may start to believe that you can eat more. During and after exercise, drink plenty of water so that you lessen the hunger signal. Do not reward yourself with food for exercise.

If you have any weight-related health issues or your body mass index (BMI) is over 30, you should consult your Doctor before you start doing regular exercise. You can calculate your BMI by going to https://www.nhs.uk/live-well/healthy-weight/bmi-calculator/ and entering your details.

Your Bonus

You can download a relaxation/hypnotic recording to aid weight control at www.hotwomencoolsolutions.com

'Losing weight helped with my menopause symptoms. I used the slow and mindful eating techniques and the hypnotic weight loss recording. I lost over 2 stone over several months. More importantly I felt better about myself, grounded and focussed. It helped me to sleep better and enjoy life.' Martha

'I haven't experienced any significant weight changes during my perimenopause but I have certainly noticed changes in my body shape. I've always been curvy, often bigger curves than I would like, but curvy nonetheless. But now my waist has definitely thickened.

I use mindful eating and the hypnotic weight loss recording to control my weight. If I put on a few pounds on holiday I know I can take them back off again using the techniques. It definitely helps me to stay healthy.' Teresa

COOL SOLUTIONS:

1. The Internal Control Panel

One way of tuning in to your level of physical hunger is to picture your internal control panel. You may have already tried this visualisation in Chapter 2 to control your temperature.

If you have been a serial dieter, you may find it difficult to recognise your current level of hunger, but the more you tune into your hunger scale, the quicker you will be able to recognise the signals from your body.

There are two techniques, the first is for you if you find it easy to visualise and the second is if you find it easier to experience signals physically.

Measure your hunger

Use the following exercises to help you tap into your unconscious mind and calibrate how physically hungry you are. Either:

Visualise a dial or sliding control with a scale of 1 to 10.

1 = 'Empty/starving' 5= 'Satisfied' and 10 = Uncomfortably full

Visualise whereabouts on the scale your current level of hunger is.

Only eat between 2 and 5 ie don't wait until you are empty/ starving or eat past feeling satisfied.

Or

Raise your arm out straight in front of you. On a scale of 1 to 10 this will indicate 5 = 'Satisfied'.

1 (hand just above lap) = 'Empty/Starving'

10 (Hand raised to a comfortable height) = Uncomfortably full

Only eat between 2 and 5 ie don't wait until you are empty/ starving or eat past feeling satisfied.

2. Spinning

Spinning is an NLP technique which uses the way the sensation of emotions moves around our bodies. Often when you crave a particular food, the feeling starts down low in the stomach and rises up through the chest into the mouth and throat. Sometimes the feeling is restricted to the head.

For you to carry on experiencing the sensation, it has to keep moving otherwise it would die away. You can use that movement by reversing it and sending the craving back where it came from.

Reduce Craving—Spinning

1. Think of a time when you have really craved a specific food

2. Replay that craving, paying particular attention to the feeling that triggers it. Notice where that feeling starts in your body and how it moves in a particular direction, and whether it has a shape or a colour. Really experience that feeling. [nb strong feelings often start low down in the body and rise upwards]

3. Imagine connecting the end of that feeling to where it starts so that you can spin it.

4. As you feel that spinning motion move it outside of your body, and spin it faster and notice what happens to the craving

5. Now slow the spinning down, and notice what happens to the craving

6. Now reverse the spin, turning it in the opposite direction. Change the colour. Notice how that feels.

7. Finally, take that new feeling back into your body and notice what has happened to that craving

Some people visualise the spinning, others find it more effective if they use their hand to emphasise the spinning motion.

Repeat steps 4-7 three or four times

3. Changing the Picture

This technique uses the way your unconscious mind decides what to pay attention to. When you picture things that are important to you, you tend to picture them closer, bigger, more colourful, clearer and brighter. Things that are less important tend to be smaller, further away, less colourful, fuzzier and duller.

By changing the picture, you can change your mind about how you feel about something. You can use this technique to reduce your craving for an unhealthy food and to increase your desire for a healthy food.

To reduce a craving:

1. Picture the food you crave. As you look at that picture notice on a scale of 1 (low) to 10 (high) how much you crave that food.

2. Start to make the changes to that picture that reduce the level of your craving, for example make the picture smaller, push it further away, take the colour out of it, and make it fuzzier

3. Notice now the level of the craving. If it is still above a 5, keep making changes until you reduce it to a 1 or 2.

To increase the desire for healthy food:

1. Picture the healthy food. As you look at that picture notice on a scale of 1 (low) to 10 (high) how much you desire that food.

2. Start to make the changes to that picture that increase the level of your desire for example make the picture bigger, bring it closer, add more colour and make it clearer and brighter.

3. Notice now the level of desire for the healthy food. If it is still below 5, keep making changes until you increase it to 8, 9 or 10.

If you have an issue with unhealthy food 'calling to you' from the fridge or the cupboard, you can make similar adjustments to reduce the influence of those sounds. To reduce the craving, you can imagine pushing the sound further away, making it softer and less distinct and changing it to a Mickey Mouse voice.

Chapter 4

HOW DO I KEEP MY 'MOJO'?

This stage of your life could be best time for your sex life. The sex may not be as whizz bang as it has been previously but slower love-making can be more sensitive and intense. You have more experience now and you have learned more along the way. You may not have to wait for the children to go to sleep or worry about interruptions any more. This can be a time for exploring and enjoying without the bother of periods and the fear of unwanted pregnancy.

There can be a perception that the changes to the hormones during perimenopause lead to a reduction in libido but actually they can lead to heightened sexual response. Responses from older women in the Hite Report support this:

"I didn't know getting older would make sex better! I'm fifty-one now and just getting started."

"I thought that menopause was the leading factor in my dry and irritable vaginal tract. My doctors thought that it was lack of hormones...but with my new lover, I am reborn. Plenty of lubrication, no irritation."

A study in 1986 (Masters & Johnson) found that women have no decline in orgasmic potential during their lives and may become more orgasmic.

If you are already going through your perimenopause and have noticed a reduction in your sex drive, think about what might be contributing to it. Factors that might contribute to a reduced sex drive are:

- Tiredness

- Stress

- Too much alcohol

- Depression

- Low-thyroid function

- Vaginal dryness

A factor that has an enormous influence on your sex drive during later life is your beliefs. If you believe that sexiness belongs to the young, thin and perfect women that you see every day on TV and in adverts, then the chances are that you won't measure up to it. However, if you believe that being sexy is about how confident you feel and the chemistry you have with your partner, then you are more likely to carry on with a healthy and confident sex life long past your menopause.

Self-image

As you enter perimenopause you are likely to notice changes to your physical appearance. There may be changes to your skin tone and texture, or changes to your body shape. The colour and condition of your hair may be changing – and not just as a result of the work by your hairdresser!

All of these changes are natural. What is important is the thoughts you have about it, the things you say to yourself when you look in the mirror. You are probably your harshest critic. Sometimes you say things to yourself that you would never say to a friend. So, start being your own best friend (see Your BFF Mirror Technique).

Confidence

We are all born confident. Babies are confident that they will be fed and cared for. By the time you reach perimenopause you will have had a range of life experiences and you may have lost some of that original confidence.

Confident people love and understand themselves. They know what they want and they think positively even when faced with problems and obstacles. This is all about getting in touch with who you are now. You may be at a stage of your life where you are changing roles and it is time to re-assess what you want in life and in your relationships. What is important to you now? You will feel more confident if you are living your life doing what is important to you.

One way of loving yourself is to treat yourself to something, for example having a massage, getting your nails done, or a new hairstyle. Visit your local lingerie shop. It's surprising how much more confident you can feel wearing new, properly sized underwear.

Remember that if your partner is a similar age, they are probably not feeling confident about how they look. Reassuring them that you find them attractive will help to re-establish your relationship as well as giving them a major boost.

Sex

Sex is good for you. It's not just about the enjoyment. Sex stimulates the hormones, releases tension, boosts the immune system, relieves headaches, and is a great form of exercise. A research project involving 55,000 respondents showed that people who had a satisfying sex life were physically healthier and more relaxed than those with an unsatisfying sex life (Institute for Advanced Study of Human Sexuality, San Francisco).

This not only about penetrative sex. There is a whole range of foreplay and intimate touch that will stimulate the production of positive hormones, improve your mood, and tone your body.

You can get back in touch with your own body and your partner's body through massage. Massage is always sensual and does not have to be the precursor to sex if you don't want it to be.

It can be a way of finding out more about what parts of the body are particularly sensuous for you and your partner. You can experiment with different types of oil, creams, and lubricants, and with different textures to heighten the experience for example feathers, fur, and ice.

If you are not currently in a relationship, or even if you are, self-stimulation is a safe form of sexual enjoyment. There are several ways in which you can masturbate using your hands or a vibrator. Whatever brings you satisfaction is absolutely fine and you shouldn't be afraid to experiment to find out what works for you.

Relationships

At this stage of your life you may have been in a long-term relationship for a number of years or you may be embarking on a new relationship. Whatever stage you are at, communication is essential to the success of your relationship generally and your sexual relationship in particular. There needs to be an understanding of each other's needs.

If you are in a long-term relationship, sex may be a subject that you have stopped talking about. You may think that you know what your partner is thinking about you and your relationship, but the chances are that if you haven't talked about it recently, you don't know what they really think. If you're at the beginning of a new relationship, now is the chance to be open and honest about what you enjoy.

So, how do you start that conversation? It's probably not a good idea to have the conversation in bed when you are both feeling tired or under pressure. Think about having a chat away from your everyday situation. You could arrange to have a date for example. Be imaginative. It doesn't have to be going out for a meal, you could have a trip to a spa so that you could both relax and have a massage or other treatment.

Once you understand each other better you can explore what works best for both of you. You might consider visiting a shop that sells lingerie and sex toys. Staff in these shops are trained to assist you and they won't be embarrassed so you don't need to be either. If you don't feel that confident you can always shop for what you want on the internet.

Pregnancy

You can get pregnant during the perimenopause. HRT is not a contraceptive and, because you may still be ovulating when you first start taking it, you could get pregnant. As a general guideline, you should wait for two clear years after your last period before you stop using contraception.

If you have been using the Pill for contraception it may have masked the signs of menopause. The Pill can be used to regulate the menstrual cycle but you need to weigh up the benefits against the potential side effects for example depletion of nutrients, lower sex drive, and decreased vaginal lubrication.

If you are in a new relationship, use a barrier method such as condoms, because of the risk of sexually transmitted diseases. There are a range of intrauterine devices (IUDs) or coils that you could consider. There is a coil which releases progesterone directly into the womb and this can help if you are experiencing heavy bleeds.

Vaginal Changes

A common result of the hormonal changes occurring during the menopause is the reduction of moisture and elasticity in the vagina. This is caused by the lower levels of oestrogen. The tissue of the vagina becomes drier, more easily irritated and broken. This can make the genital area more prone to conditions such as:

- Vaginitis – inflammation of the skin of the vagina. May be irritated by soaps, detergents, lotions, perfumes, douches, tampons, condoms, and some medications

- Yeast infections – the most common yeast infection is *Candida albicans.* The symptoms include a discharge that varies from white and watery to thick, white and chunky, pain with intercourse and or urination, and vaginal itching. Candida is present in the vagina normally but certain factors can cause it to get out of balance giving rise to a yeast infection.

- Urinary tract infections (UTIs) such as urethritis and cystitis. Symptoms of UTIs vary but can include painful and frequent urination, back or lower tummy pain, and fever.

You may not be able to prevent all vaginal infections but there are some simple things you can do to help to avoid them:

- Wear loose clothes to allow air to circulate around your lower body.

- Avoid wearing tights

- Wear cotton underwear.

- Wash your genital area thoroughly every day, and avoid using perfumed soaps and sprays

- Wipe your genital area from front to back to avoid pushing germs into your vagina

- Drink lots of fluids, preferably water.

- Urinate frequently including:
  - Before sex for comfort and to reduce the risk of bruising, and
  - After sex to flush bacteria from the urethra

- Use a water based or organic lubricant during intercourse to reduce friction.

- Avoid using biological washing powders and liquids to wash underwear.

Consult your doctor if your symptoms last for more than 5 days, you develop a high temperature, your symptoms suddenly get worse, or you have diabetes.

You might consider food supplements that help maintain a healthy vagina:

- Omega 3 Oil - to control inflammation and help to lubricate the body.

- Vitamin C – to help your body manufacture collagen to keep the walls of the vagina elastic.

- Probiotic – to aid good levels of beneficial bacteria in the digestive system.

- Cranberries - stop the bacteria that give rise to cystitis from attaching to the wall of the urinary tract. Use a concentrated dried form or unsweetened cranberry juice.

For more information about supplements see *Natural Solutions to Menopause* by Marilyn Glenville

Incontinence

Incontinence, or the involuntary loss of control of the bladder, is an embarrassing problem that can affect women at any age regardless of whether they have given birth or not. A third of all women suffer bladder control problems and around half of all women in nursing homes are there primarily because their incontinence is unmanageable at home (Chiarelli, 1995).

Incontinence comes in two types:

- Urge incontinence – where you get a sudden need to urinate and may not be able to get to the toilet in time. This condition is usually caused by an overactive or irritable bladder. Even though you may not feel as though your bladder is full, the sight, sound or even the thought of water or urination can cause the need to urinate and a release or urine. The solution is to retrain the bladder by gradually increasing the time between trips to the toilet until the bladder becomes less sensitive.

- Stress incontinence – is the most common form of incontinence and you will be familiar with this if you have ever wet yourself while sneezing, laughing, or exercising. At menopause it can arise from pelvic floor issues due to:

  o Lower oestrogen levels

  o Constipation

  o Chronic cough

  o Being overweight

  o Drugs

  o Spinal problems

  o Catheters

  o Stroke, Parkinson's Disease and diabetes

The good news is that you can put away the absorbent pads and stop feeling embarrassed because there are effective exercises that you can do that will strengthen your pelvic floor. The pelvic floor is a complex group of muscles that is generally poorly understood but strengthening them will assist with bladder control and improve your experience of sex.

You can start doing pelvic floor exercises, known as Kegels, at any age and if you are already experiencing menopause symptoms it is definitely case of 'better late than never'.

Kegel Exercises:

1. Identify the pubococcygeus (PC) muscles when you go to the toilet by feeling the muscles that contract when you stop and start the flow of urine.

2. Contract the PC muscle tightly and hold for 3 seconds, relax for 3 seconds, and repeat. Gradually build up to 10 seconds.

3. Contract and release the PC muscles as rapidly as you can, starting with 30 and building up to 200.

4. Lie down on your back, knees bent, with your feet flat on the floor. Raise the pelvis until you feel the pull and then begin squeezing.

For more information and exercises see the Resources Section

If pelvic floor exercises do not improve you symptoms or the problem persists there may be some underlying cause that needs further investigation. Do not suffer in silence. Consult your doctor about medication and treatment options.

'Sexually I have experienced a new phase in my life where I can enjoy sex, have fun with it, try out new things and to be relaxed about it. I have experimented with lots of different positions and had sex in some different places which adds to the fun and overall excitement. I have not experienced any vaginal dryness and have not needed to use any lubricants during intercourse.

At times I have felt a little self-conscious of my stretch marks and the fact that my breasts are not as pert as they used to be, and that is part of who I am. I feel sexy in myself, most of the time, although I do struggle with my sexuality at times. I feel that that is down to my

up-bringing rather than my age. I have to say that I left my marriage 8 years ago, had I still been in that relationship I do not think that I would be having a sexual relationship with my ex-husband as we had not had sex for 15 years prior to our separation! Sally

"When I put my make-up on in the morning, I smile at my reflection in the mirror so that I put my blusher in the right places. I love that my first smile of the day is for myself!" Amelia

COOL SOLUTIONS

1. Your New 'Best Friends Forever' Mirror

You can't avoid looking in the mirror for the rest of your life so it is time to make friends with your reflection and accept who you are.

Your BFF Mirror

1. Stand in front of the mirror with your eyes closed. Think of someone who loves you and whose opinion you trust and respect. Imagine them standing next to you.

2. Imagine stepping into the body of that person so that you can see through their eyes

3. Open your eyes, looking at your reflection through the eyes of the person who loves you. See what they see, all the details about you that they love and appreciate. Feel the love and good feelings they have as they look at you. Hear what they would say to you.

4. Now step back into your own body, looking through your own eyes, enjoying knowing that you are loved for who you are. Send yourself love and approval.

2. Replace your 'faulty thinking'

Our minds generate thoughts all of the time, some are good and some are bad. None of them are real, they are just thoughts. What is important is which thoughts you pay attention to.

Cognitive Behaviour Therapy (CBT) talks about automatic thoughts, that is thoughts that pop into your mind quickly and often give rise to an emotion. They are based on beliefs we have about ourselves and the world in which we live. Negative automatic thoughts can give rise to negative emotions and behaviours.

These automatic thoughts are frequently 'faulty' in that there is no evidence to support that they are true. It is helpful to identify your faulty thoughts so that you can start to change them.

Common types of faulty thinking are:

Catastrophising: Here you have a tendency to think the worst will happen in every occasion. Events which others may shrug off you dwell on and 'turn a molehill into a mountain'.

All or Nothing Thinking: This is the black or white approach with no shades of grey. So if something goes wrong on one day you might think that there is no point continuing.

Fortune Telling: This is when you predict the future - gloomily

Mind Reading: This is when you think you know what others are thinking 'They think I'm fat/old/stupid'.

Overgeneralising: This is when you think that something must be true for all time, everyone, and all circumstances. You find yourself thinking 'Everyone must...' 'No one...' 'Always...', 'Never...'

Making Demands: This is when you think others *must* do something for you, or the world *must* operate in a certain way.

Bearing the 'Unbearable': If you find yourself thinking that things are unbearable, this is very unlikely to be true or you'd probably already be dead.

Replace your faulty thinking:

1. Identify your most common faulty thinking from the list above

2. Ask yourself: 'Is this thought helpful?' If it is, accept it. If not, think what the consequence is of thinking that thought such as the emotions or behaviour that it gives rise to. Gently acknowledge the thought and let it drift away. If it comes back, gently acknowledge it again and let it drift away. Eventually your brain will get the message.

3. Ask yourself: 'What would be more helpful to think?' Repeat the helpful thought to yourself.

4. If you notice yourself thinking the unhelpful thought, replace it with the helpful thought.

You can download a 'Faulty Thinking Journal' at www. hotwomencoolsolutions.com

Chapter 5

WHAT CAN I DO TO STAY FIT AND HEALTHY?

Health issues

If you go into this stage of your life in a fit and healthy condition, there is no reason why you can't come out of the other side of it just as fit and healthy. Some of the health issues associated with menopause are more likely to be related to getting older or lifestyle issues.

There are some health issues that are specifically related to the physical changes that are linked to the hormonal changes of the menopause.

Heart Disease

The terms cardiovascular or heart disease are general terms that can cover angina, heart attack, stroke, coronary artery disease

61

and high blood pressure. Heart disease is the UK's biggest killer of women. You may be worried about breast cancer but actually as a woman you are twice as likely to die from heart disease than from any form of cancer.

Prior to menopause, oestrogen helps to protect your heart by balancing levels of 'good' (HDL) and 'bad' (LDL) cholesterol, and keeping blood vessels healthy. Because of this, there is a higher risk of heart disease post menopause.

If you have a family history of heart disease or stroke you may have an increased risk of developing heart disease. But you are not a victim of your genes. There are various lifestyle choices that impact on the risk of heart disease including weight, exercise, smoking, drinking alcohol and stress.

Hypertension

Hypertension is the medical name for high blood pressure. It becomes more likely with age. You are said to have hypertension when your blood pressure reading is consistently in excess of 140/90 mm Hg. It affects nearly 30% of people worldwide and is a frequent cause of strokes and heart attacks.

Primary (or essential) hypertension is the term used for high blood pressure that has no known cause. Over 90% of cases are in this category. Secondary hypertension refers to high blood pressure that is the result of a disease or other medically recognised cause, for example sleep apnoea, kidney disease, excess cortisol, or other hormone disorders.

Common symptoms of high blood pressure are headaches, blurred vision, nosebleeds, tinnitus (buzzing in the ears,) and dizziness. If you have any of these symptoms and you think you might have high blood pressure you may be able to have it checked at your local pharmacy. If you are still concerned go to see your doctor who may prescribe medication and give you dietary and lifestyle advice. The sooner it is treated the better.

There are actions that you can take to reduce your risk of high blood pressure alongside taking medication. Common diet and lifestyle issues that aggravate your blood pressure are:

- Salt – High levels of salt intake (in excess of 2g a day) raises blood pressure by increasing blood volume. Reduce salt in your diet by not adding salt when cooking and eating, avoiding or limiting processed foods that contain added salt (such as breakfast cereals, cakes and biscuits), and eating fresh or frozen vegetables. Check labels on processed foods for 'salt' or 'sodium'

- Alcohol – Excess alcohol can raise your blood pressure, increase your calorie intake and make you less aware of what you eat. Control your alcohol intake by drinking water to quench your thirst before and between alcoholic drinks, start drinking later, use a bottle stopper so that you don't feel compelled to finish the bottle.

- Exercise – Lack of exercise affects circulation, metabolism and weight. If you are not used to exercise and you have high blood pressure, you should start off slowly with small exercise goals and build up. See below for more advice.

- Excess weight – see Chapter 3

- Stress – Stress causes inflammation that can adversely affect your blood pressure. Reduce stress by finding a method of relaxation you enjoy such as meditation, yoga or walking. (See Chapter 6)

- Smoking – blood pressure rises transiently with each cigarette smoked. The incidence of hypertension rises if you smoke 15 or more cigarettes a day. Women who smoke are more at risk of heart attack, stroke, and peripheral vascular disease. The advice is simple – stop smoking!

Breast Health

As you enter perimenopause you may notice changes to the size, shape, and firmness of your breasts. There may also be changes to the size and sensitivity of your nipples.

Tender and sore breasts can cause some discomfort. At night, heating pads, warm water bottles, and lavender oil mixed with a carrier oil may alleviate discomfort. It is important to wear a properly fitted bra that supports your breasts, preferably without underwires.

However, the main issue for women as they enter their 40s and 50s is the risk of breast cancer. The incidence of breast cancer rises with age. The other factors that increase the risk of breast cancer are:

- Genetics - Having a family history of breast cancer, especially among close female relatives. Only 5-10 per cent of cases are due to genetic predisposition.

- Early onset of menstruation and a late menopause.

- Having children later than average (after age 35).

- Obesity.

- A diet high in sugars and animal or dairy fat.

The good news is that nearly 40% of breast cancers could be prevented by maintaining a healthy body weight, reducing alcohol intake, exercising regularly, eating less red meat, and eating more fruit and vegetables.

In the UK, breast screening is carried for women between the ages of 50 and 70. A mammogram is an x-ray carried out by compressing the breasts between two plates. It is an uncomfortable process and can be quite painful but it is over quickly and can provide an early indication of cancer.

It is important to carry out regular monthly breast examinations to check for lumps or irregularities. The indicators you are looking for include small lumps; dimples or dents in the skin when lifting your arm; reddish, ulcerated or scaly skin on the breasts or nipples; any bleeding or discharge from the nipple; and any change in nipple position ie pulled inwards or pointing in a different direction.

To check your breasts follow the steps below:

1. Stand in front of the mirror with your top half naked. Have your arms by your side.

2. Raise your arms and put your hands behind your head. Look for differences in the shape or texture of the breasts and the nipples. Check for discharge

3. Lie down with your head and shoulders on a pillow. Lift your right arm and put your hand behind your head. Using your left hand with the fingers flat, stroke the right breast and underarm using gentle circular motions. Note any changes or irregularities

4. Repeat for the left breast.

If you notice anything that concerns you, go to see your doctor as soon as possible. Most breast problems are benign, not cancerous, and early diagnosis and treatment leads to better results.

Heavy Bleeding

In the pre-menopause stage, menstrual flow can vary in length and in volume between very light to heavy and flooding. The major cause of heavy menstrual bleeding is the variation in the levels of progesterone.

If you experience frequent, very heavy bleeding (menorrhagia) over a prolonged period of time, you need to consult your medical practitioner. Heavy bleeding can be caused by fibroids, endometriosis, pelvic inflammatory disease and uterine or cervical cancer.

Heavy periods can leave you feeling exhausted and drained. They can also result in iron deficiency anaemia and you may need to take an iron supplement. Symptoms of anaemia include feeling tired, dizziness, shortness of breath, sore tongue and headaches. Use an organic iron supplement as it is easier to absorb and less likely to cause constipation than ferrous sulphate. Take vitamin C alongside the iron supplement as it is essential for absorption. Vitamin A may also benefit you if you are having heavy periods.

There are changes that you can make to your diet to help to control heavy bleeding. Reducing the amount of meat and dairy products that you consume and increasing your intake of essential fatty acids (for example linseed oil) may help with this issue.

You also need to increase your intake of water and non-caffeine drinks to stay hydrated.

Osteoporosis

Osteoporosis literally means 'porous bones'. The clinical definition is 'a condition where there is less normal bone than expected for a woman's age, with an increased risk of fracture'.

Osteoporosis isn't painful and most women don't realise that they have it until they fracture a bone after a relatively minor accident or stress. One visible sign of osteoporosis is the characteristic bending forward position that develops in older people.

The bone mass of both men and women reduces naturally as they get older but women are more likely to develop osteoporosis. In women in the peri-menopause stage, the risk of developing the condition is partly down to the reduction in the levels of oestrogen but there are other important factors involved.

Genetics are a factor. If you have a mother or father with osteoporosis you may be at higher risk of developing the condition. Women are more at risk it they have an early menopause (before age 45) or their menstrual periods are absent for more than six months due to over-exercising or over-dieting. Some medications can affect bone density.

However, as with the other health issues already discussed, diet and lifestyle can weaken or strengthen your health. In addition to the guidance given above for dealing with hypertension there are other changes you can make specifically to keep your bones strong:

- Resistance exercise – for example weight training at the gym, using resistance bands or doing household and gardening tasks that involve lifting.

- Alkaline diet – more alkaline fruit, vegetables, eggs and fish

- Limit caffeine, sugar, alcohol and fizzy drinks

- Reduce refined bran. Eat bran as part of the whole grain for example oats or brown rice.

- Food supplements – calcium and vitamin D are important for bone health. Vitamin B is also recommended (Glenville, 2011)

If you are at high risk of osteoporosis, your doctor may refer you for a bone density scan which is known as a DEXA scan. This painless procedure measures your bone mineral density and compares it to the bone density of a healthy young adult and someone who is the same age and sex as you. If the results indicate osteoporosis, your doctor may prescribe drugs (bisphosphonates, strontium ranelate, calcitonin or HRT) and give you advice on food supplements, diet and lifestyle.

Headaches and Migraine

There is a big difference between headaches and migraines, as you will know if you have experienced the latter. Headaches are painful but not usually associated with other symptoms. Migraines can be associated with a range of other symptoms including blurring and changes in vision, fatigue, nausea, and vomiting.

You may already be familiar with headaches and migraines that are related to your menstrual cycle. Some women experience migraines at the beginning of their cycle and as they reach menopause these migraines stop. Other women have migraines at ovulation or during the second half of the menstrual cycle due to insufficient amounts of progesterone being produced at this time. The same imbalance can occur during perimenopause. Migraine can also be a side-effect of HT.

Some types of food and drink can contribute to headaches for example cheese, chocolate, onions, caffeine and alcohol. You may want to keep a food journal to identify and eliminate any headache triggers (see 'Resources').

Headaches can also be related to sleep problems and stress (see Chapter 7: Can I stay happy during all this change?).

Meditation, yoga, and relaxation exercises can help to ease headaches. You may also get relief from a hot bath with essential oils such as melissa or lavender. There are a number of over-the-counter painkillers that can ease headaches in the short term.

If you are suffering from acute or persistent migraines it is important to consult your health care practitioner to confirm that you do not have an underlying health issue.

Constipation

Constipation is defined as having a bowel movement fewer than three times a week. Some people with constipation find it painful to have a bowel movement and experience bloating and the sensation of a full bowel.

You can experience constipation during the menopause due to a lack of progesterone. This reduces the movement of food through the intestines so that bowel movements become infrequent, dry and pebble-like.

There are some common foods that can dry out stools and aggravate constipation. These include potatoes, puffed cereals and toast. Apples and pears can clog your system and should be eaten baked or steamed. Dried fruit should be soaked and rinsed before eating.

Some medications can cause constipation including pain medications, antacids and blood pressure treatments. If you are experiencing constipation, check the side-effects of any medications that you are taking.

Sometimes all you need to relieve constipation is just to drink more fluids and eat more fibre. You need to drink approximately 6-8 glasses of water or non-caffeine drinks a day. Good sources of fibre are fruit, vegetables and whole grains.

Physical activity helps to keep food flowing through the body effectively. Regular exercise that includes cardiovascular and weight training activity will be most effective.

There is a specific yoga exercise that you can do to massage your colon. It is known as the yoga 'Stomach Vacuum'. This exercise strengthens the muscles of your intestines to move the waste material through. It should be practiced five times a day and only when your stomach is empty:

1. Place your feet hip-width apart and bend your knees slightly

2. Lean forward slightly from your hips keeping your back straight.

3. Place the palms of your hands on your thighs fingers pointing down towards your kneecaps.

4. Inhale deeply, filling your lungs and drawing the air right down into your belly.

5. Exhale completely, emptying your lungs so that you create a vacuum.

6. Using your stomach muscles, pull your gut upward and inward

7. Without inhaling, press your stomach downward and outward.

8. Repeat steps 4 to 7 at least three times.

Exercise

A recent worldwide study concluded that lack of exercise is more harmful than smoking in terms of your risk of developing chronic diseases (The Lancet, 2012). Exercise is anything that causes you to breathe more deeply than you normally would or causes your heart rate to speed up. Fitness is the ability to perform physical activity.

Exercise can:

√ boost your metabolism

√ help to counteract vascular damage/heart disease

√ raise your stress threshold

√ reduce obesity and the associated risk of Alzheimer's disease

√ increases the level of your feel good hormones and lifts your mood

√ boosts your immune system

√ strengthens your bones and reduces the risk of osteoporosis

√ boost motivation

√ counteract depression

√ improve your memory

√ reduce the risk of cancer

√ improve your posture—making you look younger

Research carried out in Australia found that women in the age range 45 – 60 who exercised two or more times a week reported fewer headaches, felt less tense, tired, and fatigued and had lower rates of mental symptoms of depression than non-exercisers (Ratey and Hagerman, 2009).

The effect of exercise on hot flushes and night sweats is less clear. Using your Journal, you can safely carry out your own study to observe how exercise affects your menopause symptoms. Experiment with different types of exercise at different times of the day and see what works best for you.

How much exercise?

Start by setting yourself some achievable exercise goals and then planning to achieve them. Your goals should be specific and measurable so that you can be sure whether you achieved them. A poor goal would *be 'I will have sufficient exercise every week.'* A better goal would be 'I will have at least 16 sessions of 30 minutes aerobic exercise every month.'

To control your weight and ease menopause symptoms you should aim to have some form of aerobic exercise 4 days a week. If you are starting from a level of no exercise, this may seem daunting, but the important thing is to get into a routine so that after a few weeks it just becomes part of what you do and you hardly notice that you are doing it.

The most effective exercise programme is to have a mix of cardio-vascular activity that raises your heart rate, and resistance exercise (using weights or resistance bands) to protect your bones against osteoporosis and maintain your upper body strength and muscle tone.

For cardio vascular activity (walking, jogging, swimming etc), you want to aim to raise your pulse up to 60 or 65 per cent of your maximum heart rate and keep it there for about an hour.

Metabolism

Your metabolic rate is the speed at which your body burns calories. The good news about your metabolic rate is that:

- It is not genetically determined.

- Scientific research shows that is not fixed.

- It will change throughout your life in response to what you eat and how you use your body. If you have been a serial dieter, your body will have learnt to conserve energy by decreasing your metabolic rate.

- It can be influenced by your subconscious mind.

Regular exercise will nearly double your metabolic rate. More good news is that you carry on burning calories after you finish exercising. Your body burns carbohydrates during exercise and burns fat when you stop while it replaces the carbohydrates.

Blockers and Boosters

Given all of the excellent health benefits of regular exercise, why wouldn't you do it? Most of us have some thoughts or beliefs that are exercise blockers and the first step is to identify what they are so that you can deal with them.

Boosters are the enabling beliefs and motivators that help you overcome your blockers.

Some common blockers are set out below with some ideas about what the corresponding boosters might be.

Exercise Blockers	Exercise Boosters
Tiredness	If you exercise first thing in the morning it will make you more alert during the day. Get regular sleep.
Chronic Pain	Speak to your doctor before starting any exercise programme. Think about complementary solutions such as hypnosis and acupuncture
No time	20 minutes a day would make a difference. How can you fit it in to your schedule?
Lack of clear exercise goals	Write your goals down, review your progress daily. Put your goals up where you can see them such as on your fridge door

Lack of motivation	Find an exercise buddy or join a class to keep you committed and motivated. Do the motivation technique below.
Depression	Exercise will release hormones that will make you feel better
No money	Exercise does not have to cost anything. Walking is excellent and costs nothing. See 'Opportunistic Exercise' below.
Can't find my kit	Sleep in your kit until you get into the routine of regular exercise!

Take a moment to think now whether you have any blockers. Are there any thoughts that you have that lead to you having insufficient or no regular exercise? What would your boosters be to get you past those blockers?

Some General Guidelines

- Set realistic goals, plan to achieve them and take action.

- Two 10 minute bursts of exercise every day or 30 minutes four days a week will make a difference.

- Drink plenty of water before and after exercise.

- Vary your exercise and pick activities you enjoy.

- Wait at least two hours after eating before vigorous exercise.

- Don't exercise if you feel unwell.

- If you have chest pains, dizziness or excessive shortness of breath, stop exercising immediately.

Exercise suggestions

Planned exercise:

Dancing	Netball	Yoga	Pilates
Football	Tennis	Badminton	Squash
Aquacise	Circuit training	Walking	Jogging
Athletics	Skipping	Boxing	Weight training
Gym	Zumba	Aerobics	Step classes
Spin classes	Rugby	Sailing	Swimming

Opportunistic exercise:

Around the home:

- Gardening—a bit of digging can burn off 150 calories in half an hour

- Stairs—running up and down the stairs 10 times a day will burn off 250 calories and tone the thighs

- Housework—ironing 150 calories in half an hour; vacuuming 200 calories in half an hour

- Sex—30 minutes of sex-ercise will burn off 200 calories and tone stomach muscles and inner thighs

At the office:

- Park the car further from the office and walk

- Ditch the elevator and take the stairs

- Walk to deliver messages rather than emailing or phoning

Shopping:

- Park as far away from the shop entrance as possible

- Carry the shopping to the car to burn off more calories

Walking

Walking is excellent exercise because it costs nothing and there are lots of opportunities to enjoy it every day. You can burn off significant calories through walking and it is good for strengthening your lungs and heart.

If you're new to walking for exercise it's best to work on increasing your distance before you worry about speed. So first, you want to warm up your muscles by walking at an easy pace for 5-10 minutes. This signals to your muscles that they need to call on the fat reserves. Once you are warm, the optimal speed for fat-burning is a "determined" pace, that is the rate at which you breathe noticeably but are still able to carry on a conversation. Your heart rate should be 60-70% of your maximum heart rate. Walk at this speed for 30 minutes once you have built up to this duration. This will cause your body to use fat stores for energy, build muscle and raise your basal metabolic rate so you are burning more calories all day long.

For more information about walking and calorie calculators see www.walking.about.com

My (peri)menopause started when I was 50. I had always had heavy periods but suddenly they became irregular and I was really flooding. I had to wear multiple pads and several pairs of knickers. That went on for about eighteen months and then the periods stopped.

I wanted to do my menopause naturally and I have managed to do that using complementary techniques. I have had problems with my blood pressure and I have found reflexology very helpful for that.' Rose

'Swimming, yoga and Pilates definitely help with my symptoms. The yoga feels more mental than physical. It's like a meditation. It makes me feel at peace.' Martha

'When I started working from home two years ago, I was worried that I would put on weight. I got myself into the habit of doing 30 minutes exercise on the Wii Fit every morning unless I am going to the gym. This fits in well with my working day and I've actually lost a bit of weight.

I started learning Tai Chi when I was in my thirties. I started doing it again recently. It helps to relieve stress as well as keeping me flexible.' Amelia

'When I went into early menopause I sought help from my personal trainer. My favourite exercise is with kettle bells and I have now trained as an instructor. I lost two and a half stone in weight and dropped 3 dress sizes. I went on to take part in a Spartan Race to raise money for the British Heart Foundation.' Lily

COOL SOLUTIONS

1. Set effective goals

Setting exercise goals will help to motivate you. Writing them down will increase that motivation. Sharing them with someone else will help you to commit.

Use the questions below to set out your goals. Put them somewhere that you can see them every day.

My Exercise Goals

What do you want to have happen? (stated in the positive) for example *'I want to lose weight and feel more flexible'*

How will you know when it's happened? For example:

- Target blood pressure

- Target weight

- Mood change

- Time exercised per day/week

- Other measure

What will you experience when you achieve your goal?

- What will you see?

- What will you feel?

- What will you hear?

- What will you think?

When do you want to achieve it by? Be specific.

How will you get there?

Write in the table below three activities you already enjoy and would like to do more of, or those you would like to start. How could you fit them into your life?

Activity	When can do it?	How I can fit it into my life?

2. Increase your motivation

'Swish' Technique

The purpose of this technique is to replace an unmotivated picture of yourself with a motivated picture. The crucial part of this technique is the speed with which you swap one picture for another.

Step 1   Create a picture in your mind of you being unmotivated to exercise. Make the picture as though you are looking through your own eyes.

Step 2   Create a picture of you being completely motivated to exercise. Make the picture so that you can see yourself in it.

Step 3   Close your eyes and bring back the picture of the unmotivated you.

Step 4   In the lower left-hand corner of that picture, insert the picture of the motivated you.

Step 5   Once you can see both pictures, make the small picture expand as quickly as possible to cover the big picture. As you do that make a "swish" sound. Speed is of the essence so expand the picture as quickly as possible.

Step 6   Open your eyes and close them again.

Step 7   Repeat steps 1 to 6 five times, replacing the unmotivated picture with the motivated picture as quickly as possible

Step 8   Step 8 Notice how the unmotivated and motivated pictures change. Notice how it feels when you try to bring the old picture to mind.

Chapter 6

WHAT CAN I DO TO KEEP MY MIND HEALTHY?

Just as you may be noticing physical changes during the perimenopause you may also notice mental and emotional changes. Changes to cognitive ability as you enter your 50s can be due to brain shrinkage that occurs naturally due to loss of water content.

Research has shown that verbal memory can be affected by fluctuating oestrogen levels. Oestrogen's relationship to memory and language relates to how the brain stores information. You may find that you forget common words or have problems with reading during the menopause. This is commonly referred to as 'brain fog'.

Fluctuating levels of hormones can also contribute to less efficient cognitive functions but most of these symptoms are relatively mild and transient. So, you may find yourself forgetting words or walking to the top of the stairs and forgetting why you are there, but you can minimise these effects by keeping your brain healthy and lively.

If you think that your memory loss is more severe than this, you should consult your doctor. Indicators to be aware of are:

- Disorientation in familiar surroundings.

- Inability to remember recent conversations.

- Trouble making decisions.

- Repeating stories in the same conversation.

- Confusion with simple tasks.

- Trouble learning something new.

- Trouble counting money.

Can hormone therapy help?

As the production of oestrogen and progesterone starts to falter during perimenopause, the brain's delicate balance of neurochemicals gets disrupted.

At one time it was believed that HRT could help prevent dementia, memory loss and Alzheimer's disease. Further research is being carried out in this area.

There are studies that support the use of HRT for short periods during menopause. A study by the University of Illinois published in 2005 showed that women who took HRT for ten years or less had greater brain volume than women who had never taken HRT or those who had taken it for more than ten years. In the same study, the women were tested for aerobic fitness and when those results were factored in, it was shown that exercise and fitness had a significant positive effect on measures of performance and brain volume.

If you are considering taking HRT it is important to discuss all of the benefits and the risks with your doctor.

Exercise your Mind

I've already talked about the benefits of physical exercise on maintaining your cognitive ability. There are also mental exercises that you can do to keep you sharp. It could be doing quizzes, crosswords or puzzles every day or you could try some of the following suggestions:

1. Make changes in the location of frequently used objects in your home or office. If you have to think about where you have put your tea bags or favourite pen, or hair brush it will help you to set up new neural pathways. You could just try using your other hand to move your computer mouse or brush your teeth.

2. Make changes to your daily routine for the same reason as 1) above.

3. Decide to learn something new every day/week/month. This can be something small like learning a new word every day to something big like enrolling for an evening class or taking up a new hobby.

4. Try using one of the computer-based brain exercises such as MindFit or Brain Gym.

Whatever you decide to do, you need to do it regularly – after all you don't get good at jogging by going for one run.

There are lots of different exercises that you can do to improve your memory and I have included some links in the Resources section. Neuroscientists have given us some good tips recently for those moments of forgetfulness:

- If you go somewhere to get something and then forget what it was, go back to the room you started in and try again. Apparently, physical doorways act as memory thresholds and you stand a better chance of remembering if you are in the location where you had the initial thought.

- If you can't remember where you put something, say out loud the name of the item several times. This primes your unconscious to find the object.

The Time of Your Life

This stage of your life can be one of changes in many areas:

- Relationships – you may be facing the challenges of a long-term relationship or finding a new partner.

- Children – teenage children can pose all sorts of issues or you may be experiencing an 'empty nest'.

- Parents – you may find yourself dealing with elderly parents at the same time as supporting your growing children.

- Work – you may have reached a more demanding level in your career or be thinking about doing something new.

- Finances – this may be a time when you are starting to notice your finances easing or facing the demands of supporting children going off to University or at home without jobs.

Any or all of these changes can be a challenge that you can deal with and learn from but if there is too much pressure you may experience stress. Stress can be defined as a state we experience when there is a mismatch between perceived demands and perceived ability to cope. This mismatch can give rise to positive feelings of stretch or stress depending on the nature of the imbalance.

Stress arises when you are faced with an increase in demand and the mind perceives that the resources available are insufficient to meet these. A series of nervous and hormonal processes are set into action, resulting in what is commonly described as the 'fight or flight response'.

There are a wide variety of symptoms associated with stress. You might experience:

- Physical Symptoms such as headaches, sweaty palms, sleeping problems, dizziness, back pain, neck and shoulder pain, palpitations, weight gain around the waist, and increased infections like colds, flu,

- Behavioural Symptoms such as Increased cigarette smoking and alcohol intake, a decrease or increase in your appetite. You may have difficulty relaxing and find that you lose your temper more easily.

- Emotional Symptoms such as crying, edginess, anger, worries about health, and mood swings,

- Cognitive or Mental Symptoms such as having trouble concentrating, memory problems, inability to make decisions, and loss of a sense of humour.

It could also affect your work performance through absenteeism, poor time keeping, overworking, a fall in your usual standards, sloppy work, or being more irritable with colleagues.

It is important to be able to manage your stress because your body has not evolved to deal with sustained high levels of stress, and it increases your risk of a range of life-threatening illnesses including heart disease and cancer.

Emotional Resilience

Emotional Resilience refers to the ability to spring back emotionally after you have experienced a difficult or stressful time in your life. People who are emotionally resilient are able to recover quickly from the effects of powerful negative emotions such as anger, anxiety, and depression. They are more able to keep problems in perspective and do not get easily over-whelmed.

There are certain attitudes and behaviours that make people more emotionally resilient. Some people seem to be born with these attitudes but if that's not you, you can develop them.

See the Table below for ideas on how to develop your emotional resilience. Pick one or two to try and notice the difference in your mood.

Emotional Resilience Trait	How to develop it
Acknowledging how you feel and why – you have a right to your emotions without letting them take-over your life	1 Notice your negative thoughts and how they are influencing your emotions 2 Wear a rubber band on your wrist and when you notice a negative thought arising, twang the band and tell your-self to 'Stop it'! 3 Develop positive self-talk – every morning look in the mirror, smile and repeat a positive affirmation to your-self for example 'I am feeling calmer/more confident/stron-ger every day'.

Understanding how much control you have over your life – believing that the actions you take contribute to better outcomes influences how you respond to stress in a positive manner

Recognise that you always have options. In any situation you can look for opportunities to:

i) **Avoid** the people or situations that stress you.

ii) **Alter** the situation so that it is more acceptable

iii) **Adapt** by taking a more positive approach, adjusting your standards or looking at the 'big picture'.

iv) **Accept** and don't try to control the uncontrollable. Learn to forgive.

Evaluate each option and decide on the best.

Being optimistic – being able to view the world in an optimistic light allows you to develop your strengths and resources

1 Live a healthy lifestyle

2 Set yourself achievable goals and

3 Celebrate your successes.

4 Don't beat yourself up about the things that don't go right. There is no failure – only feedback.

5 Spend some time picturing the positive future that you want to achieve and plan to achieve it

Having social contacts – those with strong social networks tend to stay happier and healthier and cope better with challenges and stress	There are lots of opportunities to build your social network: 1 Join a sports club or exercise class 2 Enrol for an evening class or day school for a subject you are interested in 3 Get involved in a hobby group 4 Contact your friends and arrange a get together
Enjoying a laugh – laughing at life's adversities helps to immunise you against stress	1 Put coloured stickers around your home and undertake to smile whenever you notice one 2 Put aside time to have a laugh every day. Have a selection of funny books and videos to choose from 3 Call a friend who you know makes you laugh 4 Join a laughter therapy group
Exercising – exercise releases positive hormones into the blood and reinforces the message to your unconscious that you are looking after yourself.	All exercise is good for your physical and emotional health. To feel calmer you could try yoga or tai chi. Walking and talking with a friend is good exercise that you hardly notice.

Connecting with your environment – noticing the things of nature around you helps you to keep problems in perspective	Take time each day to notice the things of nature around you. Go for a walk and just look around.
Caring for others – random acts of kindness to others is good for them and can make you happier	1 Decide to commit a random act of kindness every day. Could be as small as a smile to a shop worker or a compliment to a colleague. 2 Volunteer. Get involved with a charity or group or your local church.

Supplements

There is frequently debate in the media about whether you need to take food supplements to stay emotionally healthy. The argument is generally around whether you can get all of the nutrients you need from a well-balanced diet.

If you are experiencing some of the symptoms of stress it may be helpful to support your system with supplements. You could consider taking every day a good multivitamin with minerals, vitamin C and Omega 3 fish oil capsules.

Physical Exercise

Exercise is important to your mental and emotional health as well as your physical health. It helps to balance the effects of diminished hormones and can protect against cognitive decline. Exercise stimulates the production of neuro transmitters and neurophins and creates more receptors for them in key areas of the brain.

The University of Queensland, Australia surveyed 833 women between the ages of 45 – 60. They found that 84% of women questioned exercised two or more times a week and reported that they had significantly lower rates of the physical and mental symptoms of depression than non-exercisers. In particular they felt less tense, tired and fatigued (Ratey, 2009).

Exercise is also important to your brain function post-menopause. One study showed that the most physically active women over the age of 65 had a 30% lower risk of cognitive decline. This was not dependent on the intensity of the exercise but on the amount.

In order to keep your brain healthy you need to do some aerobic exercise at least four days a week. That could be brisk walking, jogging or any activity that raises your pulse rate to up to 60 or 65% of your maximum heart rate.

'I believe that it is important for women to feel good about themselves, confident in who they are and that communication in a relationship is vital. If there are children in the relationship, I believe that once they have flown the nest it can have a major effect on the relationship. So often, as in my case, we had grown apart and once the children had left there was nothing left in our relationship.

Decisions need to be made as to whether you can stay in a relationship where you have nothing in common or whether you need to move on. Both decisions are hard, and I believe that it is important that you do what is right for you and not what is right for everybody else.' Sally

COOL SOLUTIONS

1. 7/11 Stress Relief Breathing

The mainstay of relaxation, breathing techniques is to be found in abdominal breathing. It can be used as a direct stress reduction technique. More indirectly it can be used as a form of meditation, as a way of becoming calm when you feel agitated or as a method facilitating relaxation. It can also be used as a preparation for self-hypnosis.

This technique works because the longer out-breath stimulates the body's natural relaxation response. By changing your pattern of your breathing in this way, your body automatically begins to relax.

Read through the exercise a few times to familiarise yourself with it. Then, when you are ready, begin.

1. Settle yourself comfortably somewhere that you won't be disturbed.

2. Make sure your clothes are loose. Footwear is optional but if you are wearing shoes make sure they are not tight or uncomfortable

3. Sit or lie comfortably with your hands side by side in your lap or with your arms by your side, and your legs uncrossed.

4. Close your eyes.

5. Concentrate on becoming aware of your feet on the floor, of your legs and arms, wherever they are resting, and your head against the cushion, pillow or chair back.

6. Begin by noticing the rhythm of your breathing without trying to change it.

7. Once you are focussed, start to make each out-breath last longer than your in breath. A good way to do this is to breathe in to the count of 7, then breathe out gently and more slowly to the count of 11*. When you are proficient at measuring by counting you can substitute the words "calm and relaxed" on the out breath only

8. Do this about 10 to 20 times, knowing that you will relax more each time. In the initial stages it is important to concentrate on the counting. Don't let your mind wander off. Feel the welcome sense of calm gradually flow in. (Remember to count the numbers in and count the numbers out. This is the cognitive part of the exercise).

9. Become aware of how much less tense you feel, just by relaxing your breathing and calming your thoughts, so that you can recognise the feeling more easily in the future.

* If you find it easier, substitute 4/7 for 7/11. The important thing is not the number but that the out-breaths last longer than the in-breaths.

This technique is good for instant relaxation. Just do it a few times, wherever you are, if you slip into thinking you can't cope in any situation. If possible, practice this exercise 2/3 times every day until it becomes easy.

2. Three Gifts Journal

Journaling is a way of bringing to your attention the good things that are going on in your life. It's a very positive way to end the day and releases happiness hormones into the blood which help you to sleep well and primes your unconscious to notice all of the positive things in your life.

Buy yourself an attractive notebook and every night before you go to sleep:

1. Think back over the day and remember all of the gifts you have received during that time. A gift is something positive that you have experienced. It can be a very small thing like a smile, a hug or a kind word, seeing the sunrise or sunset, a beautiful leaf, or plant.

2. When you have received more than three gifts, choose the top three.

3. Make a note in your notebook of your three gifts

This is a lovely exercise to share with a friend or partner. Discuss and rank your gifts together.

3. Three Minute Break

If you are feeling stressed it can affect your sleep. It may be that you have trouble getting off to sleep or you wake-up during the night and have trouble getting back to sleep. The Three Minute Break* is a useful technique to practice to help you to drift off to sleep.

Follow these steps:

Step 1 Take a minute to acknowledge what's going on in your head. Recognise that your mind is racing and that you don't like it. It's okay not to like it, so just allow it to happen without trying to fix it.

Step 2 Move your attention to your breathing. Notice the sensations of the breath from the flow of air over your nose or mouth, down through your chest and into your stomach. Follow the breath without trying to control it. If your attention wanders, acknowledge where it went and then come back to your breathing. Do that for a minute.

Step 3 Expand your attention to your whole body and notice what is going on such as the sensations in your feet, legs, torso, face etc. Just notice them without trying to change or judge anything. Let go of any emotions associated with those sensations. This may take practice but it is worth uncoupling your experience of bodily sensations from your associated thoughts and feelings

At the end of the 3 minutes, if you are still awake, the worries may still be there but you will be able to focus on possible solutions rather than infecting them with past experiences and regrets.

* Professor Mark Williams, University of Oxford

CHAPTER 7

HOW DO I STAY HAPPY DURING ALL THIS CHANGE?

Many clients come to me because they want to be happy, but what does happy mean? There are certain key hormones that are associated with the experience of happiness:

- Dopamine - the motivation chemical. It increases our ability to focus and motivates us to take action. Dopamine levels rise as we move towards a goal and begin to anticipate a result. It is highest when we are in active pursuit of getting our most basic needs met.

- Serotonin - the feel-good chemical. It is calming and soothing. Highest when we win anything, get public recognition for a job well done, feel part of a crowd, group or team

- Endorphins – the body's natural painkiller. Can create euphoria. Endorphins are released when you exercise, make love, laugh a lot, or relax deeply. The presence of endorphins in the blood makes you feel better and can make you smarter.

- Noradrenaline – is synthesised from tyrosine. Can elevate mood

- PEA (phenylethylamine) – produces a walking on air feeling. Manufactured during vigorous exercise.

- Oxytocin – plays a huge role in pair bonding. It is the hormone that underlies individual and social trust and is an antidote to depressive feelings.

You know happiness when you see it in other people. Happy people tend to have an upright posture with their head up and shoulders down. They breathe lower in their chest and their eyes are level and alert. And, of course, they smile.

Happiness is very important to your health and wellbeing, and laughter really is the best medicine. Laughter:

- Increases the disease fighting protein Gamma-interferon.

- Increases T-cells and B-cells, which make disease fighting anti-bodies.

- Benefits the heart.

- Lowers blood pressure.

- Lowers stress hormones.

- Strengthens abdominal muscles.

- Relaxes the body.

- Reduces pain, possibly through the production of endorphins.

Happier people even live longer!

What Causes Low Mood or Depression?

Depression is not a symptom of menopause but I have included it here because you can experience it at this stage of your life possibly due to the effects of reduced levels of oestrogen combined with other life events. Although more women than men are diagnosed with depression the actual distribution by gender appears to be equal (Yapko, 1994).

There are various theories about the causes of depression. The biological theories concern the link between depression and the lack of certain chemicals in the brain. Also, the link between depression and certain physical disorders such as substance abuse, heart disease, surgery, and diseases of the kidneys, liver, and lungs (Hollister, 1983)

The 'Human Givens approach' suggests that depression arises when you experience unmet physical, psychological, or emotional needs such as the needs for shelter, safety, attention, privacy, and friendship. Unmet needs can arise from a major life event such as death of a loved one, job loss, or a serious medical problem.

If your needs are not met, you begin to worry about it, using your imagination to create bad futures. The mind/body does not differentiate between reality or imagination so it responds fearfully to both. The worries build up, and this affects sleep which impacts on energy and motivation.

These kinds of thoughts and worries can be transient, but if they persist for more than a month you should seek medical advice.

Common symptoms of clinical depression are:

- Feelings of hopelessness that lasts most of the day every day for two weeks or longer.

- General tiredness and lack of energy.

- Difficulty concentrating.

- Loss of interest in activities that you have found pleasurable in the past.

- Sleep disorder.

- Self-harm.

- Recurrent thoughts of suicide or death.

Nutrition

There is a direct link between mood and blood sugar balance. Low blood sugar can lead to you feeling down and as though you have no energy. High blood sugar can leave you feeling so energised that you can't sit down and relax.

To balance your blood sugar levels, avoid sugary foods and refined carbohydrates such as white rice, white bread, and processed breakfast cereals. Reduce your intake of stimulants such as tea, coffee, chocolate, and cigarettes as these increase levels of the stress hormones adrenaline and cortisol, which also increase sugar levels.

Some food supplements may help to stabilise your mood:

- Chromium – stabilises blood sugar levels

- Omega 3 fish oils – increases levels of serotonin

- B vitamins – people with low levels of folic acid are more likely to be depressed and less likely to get positive results from anti-depressant drugs.

- 5-HTP (amino acid 5-Hydroxy Tryptophan) – can be effective in treating depression. **Do not** take 5-HTP without your doctor's permission if you are currently taking anti-depressants.

Mobilise your resources

The good news is that you have innate resources that can help you to meet your needs. These are:

- Memory – your ability to learn and remember so that you can develop new, supportive patterns of behaviour.

- Rapport – build connections with others to gain the support you need.

- Imagination – use it to picture a more positive future and plan towards it.

- Rational mind – to think logically about the worries you have created.

- Self-observation – so that you can be objective about what is happening.

- Dreaming brain – allows you to diffuse the negative emotional arousal.

Positive Worrying

As I have already said, people who are depressed worry a lot, often ruminating over their problems at night when they really want to go to sleep.

Worrying is not a bad thing in itself. It helps you to rehearse future situations, assess risks and plan for them. But when you are in a low mood you tend to only consider the worst case scenario – Scary Street! If you live on Scary Street long enough it will have a major impact on your mind/body system as it will release cortisol into your system and stress you out.

There is another way to think about the future. You can spend some time picturing the same event but with everything going well – that is Happy Valley! This primes your brain for a positive outcome and releases the happiness hormones into your system.

Neither Scary Street or Happy Valley are real, they are just pictures of the future that you are constructing in your imagination. The only reality is the present moment.

A healthier way of worrying is to consider both possible outcomes.

1. Think about a future event/issue that you have concerns about.

2. Imagine the very worst outcome of that event. What are the risks connected to that event that could lead to it going wrong?

3. Imagine the very best outcome of that event. What are the benefits of that event? What actions could you take that would achieve that result?

4. What would be a realistic outcome between the best and the worst?

When you think about the worst case it is important to be assess the level and likelihood of the risks occuring. If the worst possible outcome of the event/issue is life threatening and is likely to occur (eg if you don't wear a seat belt you are likely to be badly injured in a car accident), then you need to address that risk. If the risk you are worrying about is very unlikely to occur (eg aliens landing and disrupting your journey to an interview), stop thinking about it.

Mood Scale

Being aware of your current mood is useful in alerting you to take action to correct if needed. Take a moment to think about what your current mood level is on a scale of 1 to 10 where 1 is 'low mood', 5 is 'OK' and 10 is 'very happy'.

If your mood is 4 or below what are the warning signs? What are you going to do to lift your mood? What have you done before that worked? What will inoculate you in the future?

If your mood is 6 or above what did you do that made that happen? What is working well in your life? What can you learn from that? Can you do it again?

It is useful to keep a Positivity Journal to note all the things that work well for you. You can download a Positivity Journal template at www.hotwomencoolsolutions.com

'My mental health is a problem; however, this is not totally due to the menopause, although on reflection it has been more of a problem since my hysterectomy. It has also been affected by an unhappy relationship that I stuck with for the sake of my children. I also have had stressful jobs which along with lack of help and support at home have had a major impact on my life.' Sally

'When my [peri]menopause began my mood got lower and lower and it started to affect my relationships. There was a lot going on in my life at the time at work and with my children. I don't like taking medication but in the end I was persuaded to go to see the doctor. He prescribed antidepressants which helped with my mood but had some unexpected and uncomfortable side-effects. In the end, I stopped taking the tablets and started using herbal remedies. My life calmed down and I felt much better.' Jayne

COOL SOLUTIONS

1. Goal Setting

Achieving goals makes you feel good because it releases endorphins into the blood which raise your mood. Goals give structure and an organised direction to your life. They help you to take responsibility for your future and make success tangible.

First, decide what is really important in your life at the moment. What do you love or feel passionate about? Using the table below set yourself goals for that area of your life. It might be in the area of your relationships, your work, your health, or they could be weight or exercise goals.

In order to be effective, goals need to be:

- Positive – what do you want to have happen?

- Achievable – start with small goals that you know you can achieve. Once you start to build confidence and trust in your ability to get things done, make the goals a bit bigger.

- Needs related – physical and emotional. What is missing?

- Timed – when will you achieve it by?

- Specific – how will you measure it?

Goal What do you want to have happen?	Timing When will you achieve it by?	Actions What will you be doing to achieve it?
Sort out my home paperwork	*End of this weekend*	• *Get all the loose bills and letters together* • *Sort the current papers from the old stuff* • *Deal with the current papers* • *File it all away*

2. Anchoring a positive state

Would you like to be able to experience a positive emotion such as calm, relaxation or confidence at any time? Using this simple technique you can. It helps you to set up a new neural pathway that is set off or 'fired' using a physical sensation.

1. Decide what positive emotion you would like to anchor, for example calm, relaxed, happy, or confident.

2. Decide where you want to put the anchor. Make it somewhere accessible and easy to remember like on a knuckle, finger joint or ear lobe.

3. Think about a time when you experienced that particular emotion really strongly. Make that memory as strong as possible by picturing what you saw, hearing what you heard, feeling what you felt and remembering the positive thoughts you had.

4. Keep making changes to that memory to make it stronger and stronger and then measure on a scale of 1 to 10 , where 10 is the strongest, how strong it feels

5. If the feeling is an 8 or more, proceed to Step 6. If the feeling is 7 or less imagine how you could make it stronger. Could you make the picture bigger, in colour or a movie? Could you make the sounds louder or clearer? Could you make your posture stronger or more relaxed? Could the thoughts be more positive? Carry on until the feeling is an 8 or more.

6. As you feel that feeling as strong as possible press firmly on the anchor point for about 5 seconds

7. Shake out your body and your hands

8. Repeat stages 1-7 three times. You have 'set' your anchor

9. Shake out your body and your hands

10. Apply the pressure to the anchor point and notice the images that come to mind and the feelings in your body. This is 'firing' the anchor.

This is a 'use it or lose it' technique. If you find it helpful, practice setting and firing the anchor every day for at least a week to reinforce the new neural pathway.

Every time you feel that pressure on your anchor point and feel the feeling, and see the image, you can enjoy that emotion knowing you have control, and wondering how much stronger the feeling gets every time you use the anchor.

3. Get the Happiness Habit

Not everyone is born with a happy attitude but there are actions you can take to become more positive. Happiness is a choice. If you decide to use your brain to scan your world for positive things you will have less resources left to look for negative things.

• Start by buying a notebook that makes you smile every time you pick it up. For twenty-one days do at least one of the following activities every day:

- Keep a record of 3 positive things every day that you are grateful for. They can be as small as receiving a smile or as big as getting a bonus at work.

- Write about a positive experience that you have had during the last 24 hours.

- Exercise for at least 10 minutes to release endorphins, improve motivation, reduce stress and get into 'the flow'.

- Meditate for two minutes (you can increase this to ten minutes when you become more experienced). Focus your mind and stop the inner conversation. There is lots of advice on meditation but two suggestions are:

  o Get comfortable, sitting or lying down. Start by focussing on your breathing. Count 7 as you breathe in and 11 as you breathe out (or 4 and 7 if that is more comfortable). If thoughts start to pop up or the inner conversation starts, go back to counting loudly in your head.

  o Get comfortable, sitting or lying down. Decide on a word or short phrase that you are going to repeat, can be anything. Focus on your breathing and start repeating your word/phrase loudly in your head. If thoughts start to pop up or the inner conversation starts, go back to saying your word/phrase loudly in your head.

- Do one random act of kindness a day –for example sending an email to someone thanking or praising them, or making a positive comment by phone or face to face.

CHAPTER 8

HOW DO I STAY VISIBLE AFTER 50?

Some women say that they felt that they became invisible once they turned 50 – invisible at work, invisible in restaurants, and invisible to men. But that doesn't have to happen and there are many more positive examples of powerful older women - ask Madonna, Helen Mirren or Goldie Hawn! It's often a case of your self-esteem.

Your experience of this stage of your life will be strongly influenced by your beliefs. We look for evidence to prove the things that we believe to be true. Beliefs come from many different sources, for example life experiences, parents, family, teachers, peers, society, books, and other media. They are powerful because we treat them as factual even though they rarely are.

Some beliefs are enabling that is they can help you to achieve the results you desire. If you believe that this is an exciting and liberating stage in your life you will have a positive experience. Other beliefs are limiting and they get in the way of the action you need to take. If you believe that your life will be all downhill after your 50th birthday, then you will notice all the things that prove that belief.

Enabling Belief	Limiting Belief
"I'll give it a try, what's the worst that can happen?"	*"I'll look stupid if I fail"*
"Mistakes are just feedback"	*"Mistakes mean failure"*
"I can ask if I need help"	*"Asking for help is a sign of weakness"*
"I can learn how to do that"	*"I'll never be any good at that"*
"With work I can achieve my goals"	*"Nothing I do makes a difference"*

You can change your limiting beliefs. One of the simplest ways is to act as if the belief isn't true. If you do that, you start to notice the evidence that it isn't true.

Another technique is to identify the limiting beliefs and create positive affirmations to replace them (See Cool Solutions).

Visible at work.

If you are experiencing frequent or intense perimenopause symptoms you may have problems in the work environment.

These can have an impact on performance, attendance and relationships at work.

It is important to discuss any specific issues that you have with your manager even if that is a difficult or sensitive conversation. If you have a good relationship with your manager, it should not be hard to broach the subject. If not, make arrangements for a discreet conversation at a time and place where you will not be interrupted.

Do not leave this conversation until you are having an appraisal or performance review interview. Stick to the facts about what you are experiencing and do not be too graphic. Be clear about what action you need your manager to take to assist you.

If your manager is unresponsive you may have to involve a Trade Union or welfare representative. Check your organisation's policies on employee health and wellbeing. There is legislation that can be applied in respect of employees experiencing menopausal symptoms for example Health and Safety and Equality Acts.

Depending on the work you do and the nature of your workplace, the sort of issues you could discuss with your manager include:

- Workplace temperature and ventilation

- Proximity to windows

- Workstation design

- Standing duties

- Changes to uniforms

- Access to toilets and toilet breaks

- Adjustments to working time or duties.

Bullying and Harassment

You may find that as you go through perimenopause you become more sensitive to comments from colleagues at work referring to your symptoms. Men sometimes refer to 'women's problems' and make jokes about menopausal women because they feel embarrassed. However, these types of comments and banter can be perceived as bullying and harassment.

If you are subject to this type of behaviour it can lead to loss of self-esteem, poor sleep, stress, anxiety, and depression. Therefore, it is important to deal with it as quickly as possible either by discussing it directly with the person or people involved or by raising it with your manager. Do not suffer in silence.

Visible relationships

At this stage of your life you may be living on your own and feel very happy with that. Or you may be on your own and hoping to find another partner. If so, what are you waiting for? Here are some steps for safe and effective dating.

Step 1 Take some time to write down the outcome that you want from finding a new partner. Ask yourself:

- When you find the right person, what will you be doing together?

- What will you be seeing?

- What will you be hearing?

- What will you be feeling?

- What would be a 'deal breaker'?

- Are you looking for a short term or long term relationship?

Step 2 Review your current strengths and resources that will help you to achieve your outcome. Ask someone you trust about your current image. Is it time to update your hairstyle or make-up? How about your clothes? You could take a friend clothes shopping or go to a big store with a personal dresser service.

If you have attracted the wrong sort of person in the past, you may need to change something about yourself in order to attract the type of person you want. All of us have things that we do not know about ourselves but other people are aware of them. If you want an insight into what they might be, talk to a friend whose opinions you trust.

If you have had problems with relationships in the past, you could consider seeing a therapist to sort things out before you start a new relationship.

Step 3 Think about your options for meeting someone new. There are too many to list them all but you could:

- Put an advert in a newspaper

- Join an internet dating site

- Try speed dating

- Join a sports club, drama club or special interest society

- Enrol for an evening class

- Voluntary work

- Ask friends for introductions

Choose the option that feels right for you, the one that is most likely to get you in touch with the sort of person you want to meet. If you put the advert in the newspaper or on the website, then you are in control of the process, you get to choose who you respond to and who you don't.

Step 4 Take action. You don't know what will happen if you do take action but you definitely know what will happen if you don't – nothing! Once you have some possible dates take a few precautions to make sure that you stay safe.

- Don't reveal information that you don't need to. If you phone your prospective date, block your telephone number so that they can't make a note of it.

- Before the date re-read any information you have about the other person. Check them out on Google, Instagram or Facebook.

- Make the first date something simple, short and in a public place for example having a coffee

- Use your own transport so that you are not obliged to travel back with your date if it hasn't worked out well.

- Set up for a friend to call you on your mobile at a certain time during the date so that you have an excuse to terminate the date if it isn't going well.

- Watch your alcohol intake. Alcohol impairs judgement and inhibition

- Listen to your 'gut'. If something is ringing alarm bells, don't question it. Make polite excuses and leave.

- Don't let your children get involved until you are serious about the new person in your life. You don't want to attract someone who is interested in preying on your children.

Step 5 Enjoy yourself. If you find your new soul mate on your first date, well done. If not, be prepared to take your time, meet lots of new people and enjoy socialising. Everyone has something interesting to offer and you may end up with lots of new friends.

'I was 48 when I started looking for a new husband. Everyone said, 'It's hopeless, they all want women twenty years younger.' But you know, I didn't find that at all. I found the secret was to be in control of the whole process. Ignore any guys who did advertise for younger women, who'd want them anyway? And advertise yourself. Make it clear how old you are so that people who reply are those who are happy

to meet someone your age. Advertising puts you in control. They are competing against other men for you rather than you competing with other women for them.

Make it clear in your ad what you want. I wanted a long term partner. Again, people said, 'Don't put that, you'll frighten them off.' It didn't, and what would have been the point of meeting guys who just wanted one night stands when that wasn't what I wanted? Okay if that's what you want, but I didn't.

Over a period of three years I had dates with fifty men. Yes, fifty. And that's just the ones I chose to meet. Others contacted me but I decided not to meet them. Most only got one or two dates, but I went out with a couple of them for three months. Eventually I met Rick, my husband, we've been together fifteen years now and it was worth every minute of the searching.' Teresa

Being Assertive

One way to avoid becoming invisible is to be assertive. Assertiveness is often confused with aggression but they are very different things.

Assertive Behaviour	Aggressive behaviour
Standing up for yourself and your rights while respecting others' rights	Standing up for yourself and not respecting others
Believing "I'm ok, you're ok"	Believing 'I'm ok, you're not ok'

Attitudes: optimistic, positive, respectful	Attitude: domineering, forceful, insensitive, prejudiced, hurtful, mistrustful
Language: 'I want', 'I feel', 'The alternatives are…', 'Let's discuss…'	Language: 'You'd better', 'should', 'you're a typical…', 'You won't…'
Non-verbal: expressive, relaxed, direct eye contact, upright posture	Non-verbal: clenched fists, finger pointing, glaring, folded arms, shouting

There are times when it is right to be aggressive, for example when you are being physically threatened, but in most low to mid- level conflict situations an assertive approach will be more effective.

If you are not used to being assertive it is a good idea to practice what you are going to say before you approach a person you have an issue with. Gael Lindenfield (2001) suggests writing an assertiveness script so that you can rehearse. There are 4 main components to the script:

- **E**xplain – the situation as you see it. Be objective, be brief, don't theorise

- **F**eelings – acknowledge your own feelings and take responsibility for them. Be aware of others' feelings

- **Needs** – be selective, be realistic and be prepared to compromise

- **Consequences** – outline the rewards or outline the consequences

A sample script for dealing with a neighbour's noisy music would be:

Explain – *"I'd like to talk over a problem with you. Your room is really untidy. There are clothes all over the floor and there are lots of dirty dishes that you haven't brought back to the kitchen*

Feelings – *"I'm beginning to feel irritated and worried that we might start to attract mice…*

Needs - *…so if you would sort your clothes, put any dirty clothes in the wash basket, hang up the clean clothes and put your dishes in the dishwasher…*

Consequences - *…I would be very grateful".*

How to say 'No'

One of the skills of assertiveness is being able to say 'no' to family members, friends or work colleagues without causing offence. Refusing a request is not rejecting the person who made it.

When a request has been made of you and you are unsure whether to say 'yes' or 'no', take a moment to consider and tune into your feelings before responding. You may be able to avoid saying no by saying something *like 'Yes, I'd be happy to do that. I am busy today but I can fit it in tomorrow.'*

If you need to say 'no', say it early in your reply so there is no misunderstanding. Keep your response short and give reasons if you want to. It is often easier for people to accept a refusal if they understand the reasons behind it. Don't keep apologising, you have the right to say 'no'.

Use positive body language when you are refusing a request. Keep good eye contact and don't smile too much.

COOL SOLUTIONS

1. Change your Beliefs

1. Start by identifying your beliefs, both limiting and empowering. Consider what this belief gives you. Be specific.

My Beliefs	My pay-offs or consequences
Eg I am smart	eg I feel confident that I can hold my own

2. Take your limiting beliefs and decide which ones you want
    to get rid of.

    a. Write out your limiting beliefs on the left side of a sheet
        of paper. Keep it simple eg 'I am stupid'

    b. Now write the opposite statement on the right side of
        the page. Write larger and bolder.

    c. Repeat your positive statements out loud 10 times,
        saying it louder each time

    d. Refer to list daily for 21 days

Limiting Belief	Positive statement

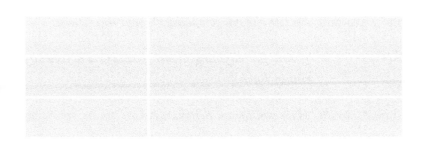

2. Broken Record

This is a very useful technique that you can use in situations where you think the other person is not listening to what you are saying or they are trying to manipulate you is the 'broken record technique'.

The broken record technique involves repeating your message and not being side-tracked by the other person. The four stage of the technique are:

1. Identify your goal

2. Make a clear statement of what it is you want

3. Respond briefly to what the other person says to you

4. Repeat your broken record message

For example, taking a faulty dress back to a shop (**broken record element in bold**)

You   *'I bought this dress here last week and the stitching has split.* ***I'd like my money back.****'*

Shop Assistant *'No one else has complained about these dresses'*

You *'I can't say anything about that, but **I'd like my money back.'***

Shop Assistant *'Have you torn it deliberately?'*

You *'No, I haven't. **I'd like my money back.'***

Chapter 9

TEN TOP TIPS FOR A HEALTHY MENOPAUSE

If you have read the whole book you may have noticed some common themes. Here is a summary of the most important tips

1. Be well informed. The better informed you are about what is going on in your body and your options for treatment, the better equipped you will be to obtain the resources you need.

   a. Keep a note of the intensity and frequency of your symptoms

   b. Use this book and other specific books and websites to understand the risks and benefits of your treatment options,

2. Eat a healthy diet. Your experience of perimenopuase and post-menopause will be significantly affected by what you do and don't eat.

   a. Eat lean protein, fruit, and vegetables

   b. Limit your intake of carbohydrates, particularly refined carbohydrates such as white bread, white rice and processed breakfast cereals

   c. Avoid processed foods and 'fat-free' or 'low-fat' foods.

3. Drink plenty of water and non-caffeine drinks. Staying well hydrated is important for your physical, mental and emotional wellbeing. The diuretic effect of caffeinated drinks (tea, coffee, chocolate and energy drinks) may flush vital nutrients out of your system. Substitute:

   a. Herb teas, fruit teas or Rooibosch (South African caffeine free tea)

   b. Pure fruit juice diluted with mineral water

   Reduce your intake of caffeine slowly to limit the possibility of withdrawal effects.

4. Exercise. A mixture of resistance exercises and cardio vascular exercise will help to keep your body and mind healthy. Exercise is not confined to organised or gym exercises. There are opportunities to exercise every day at home and at work by walking a bit further, using the stairs instead of the elevator or going to talk to someone rather than phoning or emailing.

Remember, everything that you do more than nothing could be the difference that makes the difference

5. Adopt a healthy lifestyle – it's never too late to start living a healthy lifestyle. If you give up smoking today you will start to experience the benefits within a couple of hours. Within five years your risk of heart attack falls to about half of that of a smoker. Within ten years the risk of lung cancer falls to half of that of a smoker.

    You do not need alcohol to have a good time. Reducing alcohol intake will reduce your calorie intake and help with weight control. It will also help you to control your moods and reduce hot flashes.

6. Keep your brain active. Getting older does not mean 'falling apart! Staying involved and active as you age can slow down mental and physical degeneration. Keep challenging your brain by:

    a. Learning a new skill or language

    b. Changing your routine

    c. Getting involved in a volunteering activity

    d. Doing mental puzzles and quizzes

7. Consider food supplements. Even if you eat a well-balanced diet you may experience symptoms that could be alleviated through the use of food supplements such as multivitamins or Omega 3 fish oils.

8. Sleep Well. Your mind and body perform 'house-keeping' tasks during sleep that help to balance your hormones and keep your brain healthy. Everyone is different in how much sleep they need but you should aim for between 7-9 hours sleep a night. Make sure that your bedroom is a 'sleep haven' – take out the television, computer and mobile phone. Remember, if you wake up during the night don't reward yourself by getting up and doing anything interesting – rest, relax your body and allow your mind to drift. If you must do something, have a drink of water and read something boring until sleep seems like a great option.

9. Control stress. The most important thing you can do to relieve stress is to take control of the situation. Even in the most difficult situations you always have options. Take time out to treat yourself even if it is only something small like having a five minute chat with a friend.

And finally:

10. Be positive. This can be the time of your life – but only you can make it so. If you look for the negative things in your life you will find them and convince yourself that it's all bad. But if you look for the positive things you will find them and this will be a great time for you and those around you.

CHAPTER 10

WHY MENOPAUSE IS A WORKPLACE ISSUE

In recent years much more has been discussed about supporting women during menopause in the workplace. There have been several research studies and guidance notes prepared by various organisations including The Open University, Trade Union Congress (TUC), Chartered Institute of Personnel and Development (CIPD), and Faculty of Occupational Medicine (FOM), into the impact on women employees and organisations of menopause symptoms.

Women now make up nearly 50% of the workforce and there are more women over 50 in the workplace than ever before. In 2019, this was the fastest growing demographic not only in the UK workplace, but also in America and Australia. (Brewis, J. 2019). There are 61 million women over 50 in the US workforce (Harvard Business Review, Feb 2020). There are no statistics available yet for the impact of COVID-19 on these employment patterns.

Looking at the three months January to March 1993 compared with the same time frame in 2020, the labour market participation of women in the over 50 age group had increased by 21.2 percentage points. (Brewis, J. 2020)

There are many factors that influence more women to remain in the workplace over 50. On the positive side this includes improved opportunities to progress, and changed societal attitudes. On the negative side some women feel compelled to work longer because there is a gap in women's pension provision due to the gender pay gap and the changes in state pension provision.

It has been reported that of the 3.5million women over the age of 50 in employment in the UK, 75% report that they regularly experience menopause symptoms. As a result:

59% report difficulties that negatively affect their performance

52% say they have less patience with clients and colleagues

58% experience more stress

65% were less able to concentrate

30% have taken sick leave because of their symptoms (CIPD, 2019)

Similar issues have been observed in a new study of nearly 600 working women in Japan aged 45 to 65 years (NAMS,

2020). 'Researchers in the study found that a higher number of menopause symptoms were correlated with a lower work performance. More important, they found that working in an appropriate environment (one without high levels of stress) and maintaining a healthy lifestyle helped to reduce menopause symptoms. Conversely, they confirmed that women with numerous menopause symptoms were more likely to report a lack of exercise, chronic disease, and job-related stress.'

Women are often reluctant to talk with their managers about symptoms that are having a detrimental impact on their performance due to embarrassment and to a perception of prejudice against older workers. The ease of the conversation depends on the culture within the organisation and the attitude of the manager (see Chapter 4). It does not matter whether the manager is male or female, young or old.

Menopause symptoms can affect women at any level within an organisation but it can be particularly difficult for women in senior leadership roles to talk about. They may feel that it will undermine their authority and their opportunities for progression. Dr Elizabeth Farrell, medical director at Jean Hailes for Women's Health in Australia, says, "There's a sense that somehow it will diminish their capacity to function or demean them. I think that the education of men and women about the expectations of what will happen when periods stop, and the time leading up to it, is incredibly important." (Australian Financial Review, Feb 2020).

Despite the challenges of menopause there are many positive aspects. Firstly, there is the freedom from monthly menstrual cycles which can be very debilitating. The focus can move away from concerns about reproductive issues. This is also a stage when childcare responsibilities are reducing and women have more time for their career and achieving their potential. It is like a cognitive re-boot where women can use all the knowledge and experience, they have accumulated.

Advantages of providing support

Employers who support women colleagues at menopause can achieve:

- improved productivity,

- reduced sickness leave and absenteeism,

- better staff retention

- higher morale

- improved employee relations

- a more diverse and inclusive culture

- active social responsibility

- recognition as a good employer.

Supporting women colleagues at menopause with solutions such as tailored absence policies, flexible working patterns, and low-cost environmental changes can be simple and highly effective.

Women who were supported in the workplace from their managers and colleagues reported that it was 'considerably valued'. 'They believed it enabled them to continue working well and productively.' (Griffiths et al 2010).

A major benefit to employers of taking a strategic approach to menopause and putting supportive policies in place is about corporate social responsibility. Enhancing the wellbeing of employees is not only a 'good thing' to do, it also means that the organisation will be seen as an exemplar of a good employer of women. This can lead to business awards and the ability to attract more women to the organisation as employees and customers.

The cost of not providing support

On the negative side, employers who ignore this issue make themselves vulnerable to Employment Law cases. There is employment legislation that can be applied to employees experiencing menopause symptoms. There have been several cases successfully brought by women experiencing long-term symptoms that have had a severe adverse effect on their work activities (see Chapter 8).

Approximately 20-25% of women experience disruptive menopause symptoms. A 2013 survey of 900 women in managerial and administrative occupations (Griffiths, A. 2013) found that problematic symptoms included: lowered confidence, poor concentration, and poor memory.

There are no accurate statistics for the financial impact on businesses of menopause in the workplace. A report published in 2017 (Brewis, J. 2017) considered that many of the costs of women's economic participation during menopause transitions are borne by women themselves. This can take the form of them voluntarily reducing their working hours, taking less stressful, lower paid jobs, or withdrawing from the workplace completely.

The Report, using a conservative estimate of over 174,000 women in the workplace experiencing symptoms that affect their ability to work, concluded that:

"The absence of these 174,200 women aged between 50 and 54 cost the economy at least £7.3million in absence-related costs… but this estimate failed to include other costs like "symptom-related lateness for work, lost productivity due to medical appointments during working hours [and] women who reduce their working hours due to symptoms".

Another issue in the workplace is the retention of experienced women employees. In one survey, 25% of women reported that they considered leaving work because of their symptoms. No statistics are available for the number of women who actually left.

The costs of recruitment and replacement are not inconsiderable. A report by Oxford Economics in 2014 (HR Review) estimated that the cost of replacing a member of staff on a salary of £25,000 was £30,614. This includes the cost of recruitment and the cost of lost output while training a new employee.

The business case for supporting women at menopause in the workplace is clear.

The only question is: what scale of support is suitable for your organisation?

(Extract from 'Menopause – Mind the Gap: The value of supporting women's wellness in the workplace.' 2021 by Pat Duckworth)

Resources

Menopause Symptoms Record

You can use this table to keep a note of any menopausal symptoms that you are experiencing and anything that you have become aware of that triggers the symptom. You may also want to keep a note of the stage in your menstrual cycle when you experience the symptom.

Symptom	Yes/No	Frequency (per day or per week)	Intensity (scale of 1 to 5)
Tension			
Mood swings			
Depression			
Forgetfulness			
Poor or interrupted sleep			
Weight change			
Headache			

Tiredness			
Dizziness or faint-ness			
Heart pounding			
Hot flash			
Night sweat			
Irregular periods			
Heavier/lighter periods			
Breast tenderness			
Abdominal bloating			

LINKS

You can access the following journals at
www.hotwomencoolsolutions.com

- Menopausal Symptoms Journal

- Sleep Journal

- Food Journal

- Faulty Thinking Journal

- Positivity Journal

Complementary and Alternative Therapies

For women who do not want to take prescribed medicines there is a range of complementary and alternative therapies that can help to relieve menopausal symptoms.

The best complementary therapies are holistic, that is they treat the whole person. They can generally be used alongside medical treatment but it is advisable to check with your medical practitioner if you are undergoing treatment.

When you are choosing a complementary therapist consider the following:

- Is the therapist qualified and insured?

- If you contact the therapist, do they welcome questions and answer them fully?

- Are they open about their fees?

- Do they have any testimonials on their website?

Be cautious about anyone who guarantees recovery or cures.

Acupuncture

Acupuncture can be used to remove blockages or problems with the flow of energy around the body. Various approaches are used to stimulate points around the body including the use of fine metal needles to penetrate the skin. Although the idea of needles can be intimidating for some women, most find that the treatment is relaxing rather than painful.

Typically, an acupuncturist will formulate a treatment plan after talking to the client about her specific menopause symptoms, diet, lifestyle and overall health.

www.acupuncture.org.uk

www.acupuncture.com

AROMATHERAPY

Aromatherapy involves the use of essential oils to provide a range of therapeutic healing benefits. Aromatherapy oils can be administered by inhalation or they can be combined with massage to provide benefits that range from stimulating to relaxing, depending on the individual's symptoms and goals.

There are a number of oils that can be used to provide relief from menopause symptoms including angelica, anise, basil, coriander, fennel, geranium, lavender, neroli and sage. In particular, lavender is used for its calming effect which can be helpful for stress and emotional and mental symptoms.

Aromatherapy can be added to Vitamin E oil for massage treatments and this provides moisturising properties for the skin.

http://ifparoma.org/public/findatherapist.php

NUTRITIONISTS

Food supplements can be useful in supporting health though the perimenopause, even for women who are eating a healthy, balanced diet. Multivitamins combined with minerals specifically designed for menopause symptoms are available in chemists, health food stores and on-line.

Omega 3 fatty acids are sold separately and are important for their anti-inflammatory action, helping with mood swings and in reducing hot flushes

For advice and supplements that are tailored to your symptoms you can consult a nutritionist.

UK https://www.associationfornutrition.org/about

USA https://nutrition.org/

HERBAL REMEDIES

Herbal remedies can be helpful in alleviating menopause symptoms. Remedies can be purchased in chemists and food stores but for best effect it is advisable to consult a qualified herbalist.

Women taking herbal remedies should check the recommended period for taking them as many are only suitable for short term use.

Women who are taking other medication or who seek medical treatment should tell their doctor if they are taking herbal remedies.

Some examples of possible remedies:

- Agnus Castus for premenstrual symptoms, hot flushes, and night sweats

- Black cohosh for anxiety tension, headaches and migraines

- Chamomile for sleep problems

- Dandelion for fluid retention

- Garlic for heart disease, high blood pressure, lowering cholesterol, and anti-cancer

- Hawthorn for mild high blood pressure

- Horsetail for stress incontinence

- Milk thistle improves liver function

- Skullcap calming effect on the body

- Valerian for sleep problems

UK https://nimh.org.uk/

USA https://www.americanherbalistsguild.com/

HOMEOPATHY

Homeopathic remedies can be helpful in easing menopause symptoms. A range of homeopathic products can be purchased in chemists and food stores but for best effect it is advisable to consult a qualified homeopath. The appropriate remedy will depend on the constitution of the patient and how they are experiencing the symptoms.

Some possible remedies and their indicators:

Belladonna - Hot flushes of the head and face: redness and congestion; sudden start and finish; profuse sweating of face.

Glonoinum - Hot flushes of the head and face: as above and rapid palpitations of the heart.

Lachesis - Red-faced, irritable, angry, talkative, jealous, suspicious. Worse in the morning and after sleep, from heat and alcohol and from tight cloths. Better in cool air.

Pulsatilla - Gentle and weepy, changeable moods, needs sympathy and reassurance. Worse in heat and humidity; tight clothes. Better with gentle exercise and fresh air.

Sepia - Sallow-faced, irritable, weepy, angry, depressed; loss of sexual urge; low, dragging backache. Worse in the evening, in extreme cold or humidity. Better for fresh air, sleep, vigorous exercise or dancing.

UK http://www.homeopathy-soh.org

USA http://homeopathyusa.org/

Hypnotherapy

Hypnotherapy has been shown to be effective in helping women who experience hot flushes, particularly when hypnosis includes visualisation of cool images. Women can be taught self-hypnosis so that they can take control of their symptoms. Hypnosis recordings are also very effective.

Cognitive hypnotherapy brings together hypnotherapy with Neuro Linguistic Programming (NLP) techniques, positive psychology and elements of cognitive behaviour therapy to provide treatment that can target particular menopausal symptoms including poor sleep, weight gain and low mood.

UK https://www.cnhc.org.uk/what-we-do

USA https://www.psychologytoday.com/us/therapists/ hypnotherapy

Cognitive Hypnotherapy www.questinstitute.co.uk

REFLEXOLOGY

Reflexology is based on the principle that there are areas in the feet and hands that mirror each organ and structure in the body and they are connected to those organs by energy channels. Gentle but firm pressure is applied using thumbs and fingers on those areas. The therapist can induce a state of deep relaxation and trigger the body's self-healing ability.

Regular reflexology treatments can support a woman going through menopause physically, mentally and emotionally by identifying imbalances and treating areas which need attention.

UK http://www.cnhc.org.uk/pages/index.cfm

USA http://reflexology-usa.org/

REIKI

Reiki means "universal life energy". It is a Japanese healing treatment for balancing the energy system of the body. The practitioner places his/her hands in various patterns on the body using light therapeutic touch.

Reiki therapy can be used to treat common menopause symptoms such as hot flushes, insomnia, migraines, depression and cramps.

http://www.iarp.org/

SHIATSU

Shiatsu is a massage therapy using the application of pressure on particular points of the body. Typically, pressure is applied while the client is lying down on a padded mat on a flat floor. The goal of shiatsu is to bring back the free flow of chi so that the body can come back into balance.

Prior to treatment, the practitioner will assess the client's symptoms, diet lifestyle and overall health. The effects of the treatment can be very calming and relaxing.

http://www.cnhc.org.uk/therapists/shiatsu-practitioners.htm

REFERENCES

www.nhlbi.nih.gov/whi/beckground.htm Women's Health
Initiative

http://www.figo.org/news/losing-weight-may-reduce-
symptoms-menopause-0010242 *Losing weight may reduce
symptoms of menopause.*

http://blogs.plos.org/obesitypanacea/2011/06/22/does-weight-
loss-influence-vitamin-d-levels/ *Does weight loss influence
vitamin D levels? Travis Saunders, 2011*

http://www.sciencedaily.com/releases/2010/07/100713215202.
htm

www.uq.edu.au/news/index.html?article=24445 *'Research allows
doctors to predict menopause symptoms.'*

http://www.nejm.org/doi/full/10.1056/NEJMoa030311 2003,
'Effects of Estrogen plus Progestin on Health-Related Quality of Life'

http://www.empowher.com/menopause/content/weight-
loss-not-exercise-helps-night-sweats-and-hot-flashes-during-
menopause?page=0,0 *'Weight Loss, Not Exercise, Helps With
Night Sweats and Hot Flashes During Menopause'*

www.thelancet.com/series/physical-activity *'Physical Activity'* 2012

Achor, Shawn. *The Happiness Advantage*, 2010, The Random
House Group

Chiarelli, Dr Pauline, *Women's Waterworks – curing incontinence,* 1995 Khera Publications Ltd

Foxcroft, L., 2009, *Hot Flushes, Cold Science,* Granta Publications

Glenville, Dr Marilyn, *Natural Solutions to Menopause,* 2011, Rodale

Glenville, Dr Marilyn, *Fat Around the Middle,* 2006, Kyle Cathie Ltd

Gluck, Dr Marion and Edgson, Vicki, *It must Be My Hormones,* 2010, Penguin

Goodwin, J., 2012 *What Causes Hot Flashes, Anyway?* HealthDay News, April 12 2012

Hamilton, Dr David R., 2009, *How Your Mind Can Heal Your Body,* Hay House

Harcombe, Z 2011 *Stop Counting Calories & Start Losing Weight,* Columbus Publishing Ltd

Hite, Sheer, *The Hite Report: A nationwide Study of Female Sexuality,* 1981, new York:Dell

Hollister, L. (1983), *'Treating depressed patients with medical problems'*

Lindenfield, Gael *'Assert Yourself'* 2001, Clays Ltd

Masters & Johnson, *Sex and Ageing – Expectations and Reality,* 1986

Mosconi, Lisa, 2019, *How Menopause Affects The Brain, https://www.ted.com/talks/lisa_mosconi_how_menopause_affects_the_brain/*

Ratey, Dr John J. and Hagerman, E. 2009 *Spark!* Quercus

Russell, J. 2005 *Can a vagina really buy a Mercedes? What can your pelvic floor do for you?*

Useful Websites

Continence:

ACA Association for Continence Advice www.aca.uk.com

ACPWH Association of Chartered Physiotherapists in Women's Health www.womentsphysio.com

Exercise:

Couch to 5K Staged exercise programme for new runners. http://www.nhs.uk/Livewell/c25k/Pages/couch-to-5k.aspx

Food Supplements

Advice on food supplements and women's health issues: http://www.naturalhealthpractice.com/

Hypertension

American Society for Hypertension http://www.ash-us.org/

British Hypertension Society http://www.bhsoc.org/default.stm

Hypnotension TM – complementary approach to tackling high blood pressure: http://www.hypnotension.com/

NHS UK http://www.nhs.uk/conditions/Blood-pressure-(high)/Pages/Introduction.aspx

OSTEOPOROSIS:

NHS UK http://www.nhs.uk/Conditions/Osteoporosis/Pages/Introduction.aspx

National Osteoporosis Society in UK http://www.nos.org.uk/

National Osteoporosis Foundation USA http://www.nof.org/

PERIMENOPAUSE

UK http://www.nhs.uk/Conditions/Menopause/Pages/Introduction.aspx

US www.WebMD.com/menopause

US www.fda.gov/womens/menopause

GENERAL MENOPAUSE WEBSITES:

For up to date advice and resources www.shmirshky.com

The Change Explained https://www.facebook.com/AlisonDotBrown

The North American Menopause Society http://www.menopause.org/

Information about symptoms and treatment options http://www.menopausematters.co.uk/

ABOUT THE AUTHOR

Pat Duckworth is a Women's Wellbeing Strategist, Author and International Public Speaker. After over 30 years working in the public and voluntary sector at a Senior Management Level, she retrained as a therapist and coach.

Pat works with employers who are committed to supporting employees at menopause. She provides workshops, training, and other resources tailored to the needs of the organisation.

Pat is the host of the weekly 'Hot Women Rock Radio Show: Empowering women leaders at menopause' on www.talkradio.nyc. She has published five books including the Award-winning 'Hot Women, Cool Solutions: How to control menopause symptoms using mind/body techniques.' Her latest book, 'Menopause: Mind the Gap - the value of supporting women's health in the workplace' was published in January 2021 and has been highly acclaimed.

Pat makes the subject of menopause accessible and provides practical advice for women leading a busy, modern life.

You can see more at www.patduckworth.com

Books by Pat Duckworth:

Cool Recipes for Hot Women https://www.amazon.co.uk/Cool-Recipes-Hot-Women-Duckworth/dp/099266201X/

How to Survive Her Menopause https://www.amazon.co.uk/How-Survive-Her-Menopause-Practical/dp/0992662001/

Hot Women Rock https://www.amazon.co.uk/Hot-Women-Rock-discover-entrepreneurial/dp/0992662028/

Menopause: Mind the Gap https://www.amazon.co.uk/Menopause-supporting-womens-wellness-workplace-ebook/dp/B08R7SLMWJ/